Clinical Tests

Renal Disease

Dr P. Sweny MD FRCP
Senior Lecturer and Hon Consultant

Dr Z. Varghese MSc PhD
Associate Director Renal Research Unit

Department of Nephrology and Transplantation
The Royal Free Hospital
London

Wolfe Medical Publications Ltd

While every effort has been made to ensure that all drug dosages and histochemical values are correct, no liability can be accepted by the authors or publishers for any error.

Copyright © P. Sweny, Z. Varghese, 1988
Published by Wolfe Medical Publications Ltd, 1988
Printed by Royal Smeets Offset b.v., Weert, The Netherlands
ISBN 0 7234 0873 4

This book is one of the titles in the series of
Wolfe Medical Atlases, a series that brings together
probably the world's largest systematic published
collection of diagnostic colour photographs.
    For a full list of Atlases in the series, plus forthcoming
titles and details of our surgical, dental and veterinary
Atlases, please write to Wolfe Medical Publications Ltd,
2-16 Torrington Place, London WC1E 7LT.
General Editor, Wolfe Clinical Tests Series:
D. Geraint James, MA, MD, FRCP (Lond)

Already published in this series
Histopathology
Geriatric Medicine

CONTENTS

Preface

There are many ways to investigate kidney structure and function. Some tests have remained the province of physiologists and not gained acceptance in clinical nephrology. Such tests are not discussed in detail as the purpose of this book is to help clinicians caring for patients with renal disease. Where possible instructions are given for carrying out the simpler tests. References to more detailed laboratory techniques are given at the end of the book, and references have also been given for most of the more common tests of renal function.

Somewhat arbitrarily the book is divided into sections dealing with progressively more detailed and complex tests. It is of course not necessary to investigate all patients in the order set out in the book, which is merely a guide. With experience clinicians will select what they consider to be the most helpful tests. This book aims to discuss the range of tests available and indicate where they will be most helpful.

Acknowledgements

The authors would like to thank the following and their Departments for providing many of the Illustrations used in this book:

Dr R. Dick	Radiology *
Dr L. Berger	Radiology*
Dr A. Hilson	Nuclear Medicine *
Dr I.P. Beswick	Histopathology *
Dr M. Chappel	Histopathology *
Miss J. Lewin	Histopathology *
Dr R. Irving	Lewisham District General Hospital
Dr S.B. Rosalki	Chemical Pathology *
Dr P. Collinson	Chemical Pathology *
Dr J. Hunter	St. Thomas' Hospital
Mr C.C. Gilson	Medical Illustration *
Dr A. Rees	Hammersmith Hospital
Dr D.F. Birch	Melbourne, Australia
Dr P. Noone	Royal Free Hospital *
Dr M. Raftery	Nephrology and Transplantation *

* Royal Free Hospital and School of Medicine

We would also like to thank Dr K. Farrington for much helpful advice and criticism.

List of Tables: page

List of Figures:

1: INTRODUCTION

As with the investigation of any medical problem, the tests used in renal disease are selected after a sound base has been provided by a careful history and full physical examination. Investigations must serve several different purposes, not only diagnosis (Table 1). Not only can impaired renal function affect the function of many other organs and systems, but the kidney may also be involved as part of another disease in one of the multisystem diseases (e.g. systemic lupus erythematosus and diabetes mellitus). In trying to define the priorities, three principal questions confront the clinician, although more may be asked later (Table 2):
1. Is renal function impaired?
2. Is there obstruction to the flow of urine?
3. Is the disease acute or chronic?

Is renal function impaired?

The kidney has several important functions which can all be assessed by appropriate tests (Table 3). The two most important biochemical assessments that have to be made are whether the elimination of nitrogenous waste products is adequate (glomerular filtration) and whether essential molecules are being retained (the integrity of the glomerular filtration barrier and tubular reabsorption). The balance between the production of nitrogenous waste products and their elimination by the kidney is reflected in the plasma urea or, better still, by the plasma creatinine concentration. More formal estimates of glomerular filtration rate (GFR) can be made from the creatinine clearance or, more accurately, from the clearance of isotopically labelled EDTA (^{51}CrEDTA). The presence of protein and red cells in the urine may suggest glomerular damage, particularly if proteinuria is in excess of 2g/24 hrs. and if the red cells are present as dysmorphic red cells or as red cell casts. Tubular dysfunction is suggested by inappropriate leaks such as glycosuria, aminoaciduria or phosphaturia. An inability to produce an acid urine or a concentrated urine or the appearance of low molecular weight proteins in the urine may also suggest tubular damage.

Is there obstruction of the renal tract?

Obstruction to the free drainage of urine can occur at any level from the nephron down to the external urinary orifice. Prolonged obstruction produces progressive renal damage. It is therefore vital to exclude obstruction early in the course of investigation so that the opportunity for curative surgical treatment is not lost. The hallmark of obstruction is dilatation of the collecting system and ureter, which can be readily demonstrated by ultrasound or by contrast radiology.

Is the disease acute or chronic?

Acute disease offers the possibility that the pathological process can be halted and reversed, restoring normal renal function. Chronic disease implies irreversible scarring, and the best that can be offered the patient is treatment aimed at delaying further deterioration. A sense of urgency must accompany the investigation of acute renal disease. Small kidneys imply chronic disease as do the presence of anaemia and metabolic bone disease (Table 4).

Progressive investigation of patients with suspected renal disease

Against the background of the various questions that have to be asked about the patient with suspected renal disease, a logical system of investigation can be devised. It is sensible to group investigations into initial, intermediate and specialised tests (Table 5). The initial screening tests will define whether or not the patient does have renal disease. The intermediate tests define the basic anatomy and the extent of functional impairment of the kidneys. The relevant specialised tests can then be selected to define precisely what is going on.

Table 1: The purposes of investigation

1 Diagnosis:
    (a) Choice of treatment
    (b) Prognosis

2 Evidence of complications secondary to impaired kidney function

3 Monitoring:
    (a) Progression or activity of the underlying disease
    (b) Response to treatment
    (c) Detection of acute-on-chronic renal disease.

Table 2: Diagnostic questions

QUESTION	TEST
Impaired function	Plasma creatinine and creatinine clearance 24-hour urine protein excretion Tubular leaks
Obstruction	Ultrasound or intravenous urogram Antegrade pyelogram
Acute or chronic disease	Kidney size
Inflammation	Urine microscopy for cells and casts Tubular enzymes in urine
Infection	Culture
Neoplasia	Radiology Cytology Biopsy
Impaired production of hormones	Erythropoietin: anaemia $1,25-(OH)_2D_3$: bone disease
Impaired response to hormones	ADH: polyuria PTH: hypophosphaturia and reduced nephrogenic cyclic AMP Aldosterone: hyperkalaemia and acidosis

Table 3: Functions of the kidney

FUNCTION	SITE
Elimination of nitrogenous waste products	Glomerular filtration
Retention of macromolecules	Glomerular filtration barrier

Reclamation of essential molecules:
    Sodium
    Bicarbonate
    Phosphate
    Glucose
    Amino acids
    Potassium
	Proximal tubule

Control of urine concentration:
    Dilution-concentration
        +
    Free water clearance
	Ascending limb of the Loop of Henlé and
	Collecting ducts

Acidification of urine:
    Bicarbonate reclamation
    H^+ secretion
	Proximal tubule
	Distal tubule

Hormone production:
    Erythropoietin
    $1,25-(OH)_2D_3$
	Site uncertain
	Mitochondrial site
	Cell type not known

Renin production	Juxtaglomerular apparatus
Catabolism of polypeptide hormones	Proximal tubule

Table 4: Acute or chronic renal failure

	ACUTE RENAL FAILURE	CHRONIC RENAL FAILURE
History:	Clear precipitating event	Insidious onset
Examination:	Often normal	Pallor Pigmentation Peripheral neuropathy Growth retardation Skeletal deformity
Investigation:	Normal or large kidneys Normal haemoglobin No evidence of osteodystrophy	Small kidneys Anaemia Biochemical evidence of bone disease

Table 5: Progressive investigation of patients with suspected renal disease

1 Initial investigations
Urine stick test: blood
                                      protein
                                      glucose
                                      pH

Urine microscopy: cells
                                      casts

Plasma: urea
                                      creatinine
                                      electrolytes: sodium
                                                     potassium
                                                     chloride
                                                     bicarbonate
                                                     calcium
                                                     phosphate

Mid-stream urine for culture

2 Intermediate investigations:
Ultrasound
Plain X-ray of renal tract: kidney, ureter, bladder (KUB)
Intravenous urogram (IVU)
24-hour urine collection: creatinine clearance
                          protein excretion

3 Specialised investigations:
Further radiology
Isotope scans
Specialised renal tubule function tests
Biopsy
Endoscopy
Tests for multisystem diseases

2: INITIAL INVESTIGATIONS

Macroscopic appearance of urine

Careful inspection of a fresh specimen of urine may be helpful (Table 6). The concentration of urine cannot be judged by colour. Urine is dark because of the presence of a number of pigments (urochromes) and not because of the amount of excreted solutes. Urine may be cloudy because of phosphates and not necessarily infected. Red urine may be due to drugs, not blood. Red cells produce a characteristic smoky appearance of the urine. If froth persists after shaking, this suggests proteinuria. Urine that is milky after meals but which clears after an overnight fast suggests the presence of chyluria.

Urine dip sticks

A variety of commercially supplied sticks is available.

It is important that the manufacturers' instructions are strictly adhered to. Old sticks should be discarded. It is preferable to test a fresh early morning specimen of urine so that dilution artefacts do not occur. At a minimum, urine should be tested for pH, glucose, blood and protein (1).

pH

Normal urine is slightly acidic but can vary between pH 4.5 to 8 with changes in diet. If an early morning urine has a pH of less than 5.3 there is unlikely to be a significant defect in urinary acidification. It is worth remembering that urea-splitting micro-organisms produce a persistently alkaline urine.

Blood

The orthotolidine reagent strip is specific for red cells, free haemoglobin and myoglobin. These iron porphyrin pigments catalyse the oxidation of orthotolidine to a blue product by oxygen released from hydrogen peroxide (1).

Sensitivity: $\geq$ 10,000 red cells per millilitre of urine. Macroscopic haematuria occurs at 0.5 ml. blood/litre of urine.

Errors: False positives will occur if the urine contains oxidising agents, and false negatives if the urine contains reducing agents, e.g. ascorbic acid. Small numbers of red cells can only be detected by microscopy.

Table 6: Macroscopic appearance of the urine

APPEARANCE	CAUSE
Milky	Acid urine: urate crystals Alkaline urine: insoluble phosphates Infection – pus Spermatozoa Chyluria
Smoky pink	Haematuria (> 0.5 ml/l)
Foamy	Proteinuria
Blue/Green	Pseudomonas urinary tract infection Santonin Bilirubin Methylene blue
Pink/red	Aniline dyes in sweets Porphyrins (on standing) Blood, haemoglobin, myoglobin Drugs, e.g. phenindione, phenolphthalein Anthocyanins (beetroot)
Orange	Drugs: anthraquinones (laxatives) rifampicin Excess urobilinogen
Yellow	Mepacrine Conjugated bilirubin Phenacetin Riboflavin
Brown/black	Melanin (on standing) Myoglobin (on standing) Alkaptonuria
Green/black	Phenol Lysol
Brown	Drugs: phenazopyridine, furazolidone, L-dopa, niridazole Haemoglobin and myoglobin (on standing) Bilirubin

A positive stick test should be confirmed by microscopy of the urine deposit as both intact red cells and free haemoglobin (or myoglobin) give a positive result. If red cells are not seen on microscopy, urine should be tested for myoglobin and haemoglobin, as described in Chapter IV, Section 6. Stick tests cannot be used as a substitute for microscopy.

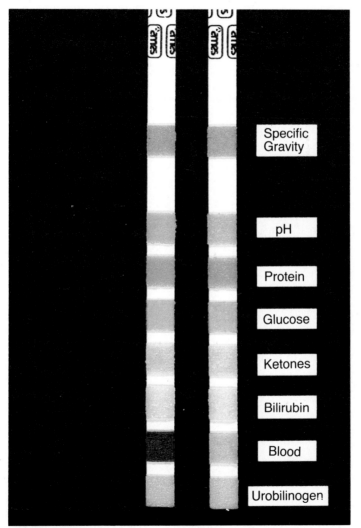

1 Urine dip sticks

Protein

The dip stick measures the urine protein by altering the colour produced by tetrabromphenol blue, the so-called 'protein error method'. Briefly, tetrabromphenol blue is yellow at pH3 and changes to a blue-green colour at pH4. The blue-green colour will appear at pH3 when protein is present (1). Protein produces a shift in the pH optimum of the indicator dye. The protein concentration should be read immediately after removing the stick from urine as the reagent strip contains a citrate buffer which maintains the pH of the paper at about pH3.

Sensitivity: $\geq$ 300 mg/1.

Errors: Free light chains (Bence-Jones Protein) are not readily detected by the stick test. A very dilute specimen may also give a false negative. False positives occur with very alkaline urine and with very concentrated samples. If the stick is left to soak in urine or there is a marked delay in reading the strip, then false positives can occur.

A positive stick test should be confirmed by a 24-hour urine collection with precise chemical quantitation of the total daily urinary protein excretion.

Although proteinuria is one of the cardinal features of renal disease, several important diseases may not be associated with protein in the urine, e.g. obstruction and chronic pyelonephritis. Proteinuria in excess of 2g per 24 hours is almost always indicative of an underlying glomerular lesion.

Osmolality

Sticks are available that determine osmolality, although it is more accurately measured by the depression of freezing point. If the early morning urine osmolality is above 800mOsm/kg. then the patient can probably concentrate his urine normally. Osmolality is to be preferred to

Table 7: Comparison between osmolality and specific gravity (SP.GR.)

MOSMOL/KG	SP.GR.
100	1.003
200	1.006
350	1.010
400	1.012
600	1.018
800	1.024
1,000	1.030
1,200	1.036

the older measurement of specific gravity (Table 7). Osmolality measures the number of particles per kg of the solvent. It expresses the sum of the moles of all electrolytes and other undissociated molecules per kg of the solvent. Specific gravity is a measure of the total weight of dissolved substances (osmolarity expresses the number of particles per litre of solution). Protein and glucose increase specific gravity more than they increase osmolality because they are dense particles. What is required in clinical practice is an index of the quality of urine which is best reflected by the number of particles present per kg of solvent, i.e. osmolality rather than specific gravity.

Nitrite Test

Nitrites can be demonstrated in the urine by the use of a diazotisation reaction in which nitrite in the urine provides the basis for the formation of a diazonium compound from a precursor such as para-arsanilic acid. This diazonium compound then complexes with a suitable substance (N-1-naphthylethylenediamine) to form a pink-coloured product.

In the presence of infection urinary nitrate derived from the diet may be converted to nitrites. Over 90% of the common urinary pathogens are nitrite-forming bacteria.

False positives occur if bacterial overgrowth is allowed to develop during delayed transit before testing. False negatives occur in patients on ascorbic acid or if frequent voiding of dilute urine does not allow sufficient time for nitrites to be produced. The test is a useful screening procedure for infection.

Glucosuria

The stick test for the detection of glucose is based on a specific enzyme (glucose oxidase) which releases hydrogen peroxide from glucose. The hydrogen peroxide then oxidises an indicator substance to produce a graded colour change. This test is therefore specific for glucose and will not detect other sugars such as pentose, galactose or fructose. Large doses of ascorbic acid block the reaction. A positive stick test for glucose must be interpreted in relation to the plasma glucose level. If there is a tubular defect in the reabsorption of glucose, then glucosuria occurs in the presence of a normal plasma glucose.

Leucocyte esterase test

Esterases specific for leucocytes will convert an indoxyl ester substrate into indoxyl in the presence of air to produce a blue colour. Appropriate sticks have recently been introduced. The test accurately detects the presence of viable leucocytes in the urine and will also detect the esterases released from degenerated cells.

Urine microscopy

Urine microscopy is an essential part of the evaluation of the patient with suspected renal disease. It should not be delegated to a busy microbiology laboratory, nor to an inexperienced junior doctor or medical student. Careful microscopy can be diagnostic and save valuable time and unnecessary investigations. Normal urine contains few cells or casts (Table 8). However, intercurrent fever or recent physical exercise will increase the number of cells and casts found in the urine. A fresh early morning urine sample after a night's rest is the best specimen to examine. Potent diuretics, such as frusemide, can also increase the excretion of some cells and casts.

Method

A clean, fresh mid-stream sample of early morning urine is collected. A few drops of acetic acid (5–10% v/v) are added if necessary to reduce the urine pH to 6 or less to prevent precipitation of phosphates. Ten millilitres of urine is centrifuged in a conical test tube at about 1,500rpm (750g) for three to five minutes. The supernatant is decanted and the sediment gently resuspended in 0.5ml. of urine. One drop is then placed on the microscope slide and examined by light microscopy. A good phase contrast microscope is ideal but an ordinary light microscope will suffice. Semi-quantitative counts of cells and casts are made and expressed as numbers seen per low power field or per high power field (2–8). One or two drops of a modified Sternheimer's stain (e.g. Sedi-stain ®) may be added to the resuspended deposit to aid differentiation of tubular cells from polymorphs.

Casts, particularly red cell casts, are somewhat fragile and may be disrupted by rough handling and degenerate on storage. To aid their detection 20ml. of urine can be filtered through a 5μm Millipore® filter and the filter with its retained casts stained with Papanicolaou's stain.

Interpretation of Results

Red Cells: The presence of red cells in the urine confirms that haematuria, detected by stick testing, is not due to free haemoglobin or myoglobin. Dysmorphic red cells may be identified by phase contrast microscopy (2). They indicate that the bleeding into the urinary tract is occurring at the level of the glomerulus as the red cell membrane is damaged on traversing the glomerular filtration barrier. If more than 70% of the cells are dysmorphic, glomerular bleeding is to be suspected. Urine from normal individuals contains small numbers of dysmorphic cells, suggesting that

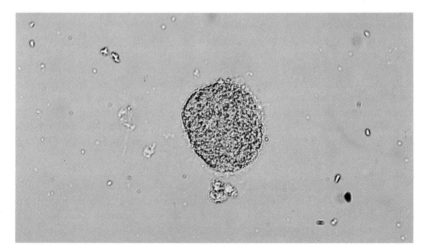

2 Phase contrast microscopy of urine sediment: Dysmorphic red cells of glomerular bleeding. Note the variation in the appearance of the red cells. In lower urinary tract bleeding the great majority of the red cells appear similar (isomorphic) and such patients require detailed urological investigation.

3 Oval fat body. These are tubular cells laden with lipid droplets and are typical of the nephrotic syndrome.

the few red cells present in normal urine enter at the glomerulus. The finding of normal (isomorphic) cells in the urine suggests that a 'surgical' cause for the haematuria is present. It is important that haematuria is always fully investigated (Chapter 8).

Tubular epithelial cells: These cells are shed into the urine in large numbers in acute tubular necrosis from nephrotoxic agents or acute ischaemia. When laden with lipid droplets in the nephrotic syndrome, they produce oval fat bodies (3).

Leucocytes: The presence of large numbers of polymorphonuclear leucocytes suggests infection. If large numbers of bacteria and polymorphs are seen on a fresh specimen of urine, then infection is likely to be present. If doubt exists in differentiating leucocytes from tubular epithelial cells, a few drops of 5% acetic acid can be added to the urinary sediment. This dissolves intracytoplasmic granules, revealing the shape of the nuclei to aid differentiation. Stains such as Sedi-stain℗ are also helpful. Large numbers of leucocytes in the absence of infection (sterile pyuria) are seen in analgesic nephropathy, stones, renal tuberculosis and in an inadequately treated urinary tract infection.

Squamous epithelial cells: These cells are shed from the bladder and urethra and are a normal finding in urine. Too many obscure the more important cells and casts in the urine. Their presence in large numbers represents inadequate sample collection.

Casts: Casts are formed from a proteinaceous matrix of Tamm-Horsfall protein, which is secreted into the tubular lumen. The casts appear in the urine as cylindrical structures, having been washed out from the nephron. They decay with time and may be broken up by shaking or too vigorous centrifugation as well as alkalinisation of the urine. Depending on the appearance and the cells embedded in the cast, different types may be recognised.

Red cell casts: If red cells are embedded in a cast it implies that the bleeding is occurring at the glomerular level. Red cell casts are highly suggestive of glomerulonephritis and should not be missed because they indicate that the haematuria is originating from within the kidney (4). They are also sometimes seen in conditions not strictly termed glomerulonephritis, such as accelerated phase hypertension and the haemolytic uraemic syndrome. Patients with allergic tubulo-interstitial nephritis may also have occasional red cell casts in the urine.

Leucocyte casts: Acute bacterial pyelonephritis produces leucocyte casts. They may also sometimes be found in patients with an acute proliferative exudative glomerulonephritis and in patients with acute tubulo-interstitial nephritis.

Tubular epithelial cell casts: Intrarenal inflammation and tubular damage produces tubular epithelial cell casts. They are found in both glomerulonephritis and in acute tubular necrosis (5). Fatty casts are found when the tubular cells are laden with lipid droplets, as in the nephrotic syndrome.

Hyaline casts: These are structureless, transparent casts composed of Tamm-Horsfall protein which is secreted by the ascending limb of the loop of Henlé and the distal convoluted tubule (6). A few may be found in normal urine, and they increase in number during fever and after exercise.

Granular casts: The granules are thought to be protein aggregates rather than the product of degenerated cells (7). They may be found in normal urine and after exercise, but large numbers suggest parenchymal renal damage.

Broad waxy casts: These casts are found in chronic renal failure. They are formed in the few remaining dilated hypertrophied nephrons, hence their broad diameter.

Table 8: Normal urine microscopy

CELLS AND CASTS	MICROSCOPY	EXCRETION RATE/ 12 HOURS
Leucocytes	1 – 2 per HPF	300,000
Erythrocytes	1 per 2 – 3 HPF	25,000
Tubular cells	1 per 10 HPF	–
Hyaline casts	1 per LPF	1,000
Granular casts	1 per LPF	500 – 1,000

HPF = High power field ($\times$ 40 objective)
LPF = Low power field ($\times$ 10 objective)

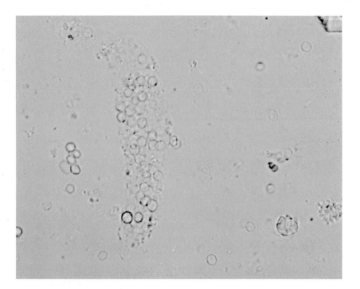

4   Red cell cast

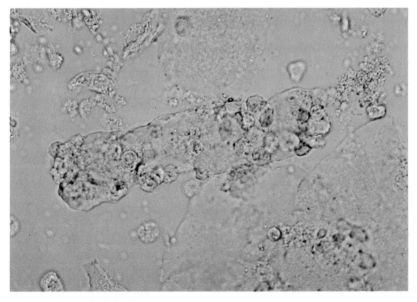

5   Tubular epithelial cell cast

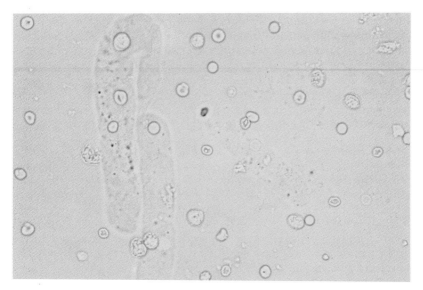

6   Red cells, tubular epithelial cells and hyaline casts

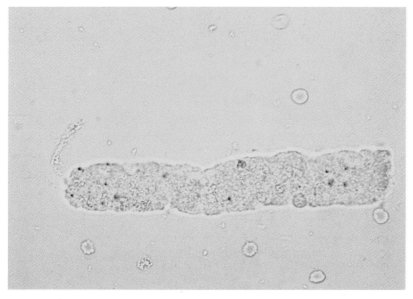

7   Granular casts

Pigment casts: Haemoglobin and myoglobin are filtered by the glomerulus and may contribute to the formation of casts. They have a characteristic honey colour and are sometimes referred to as 'brown sugar' casts.

Crystals: There is little value in defining the crystals in urine in great detail as they are so dependent upon urine concentration and pH. The one major exception to this general rule is the identification of the flat hexagonal crystals which are typical of cystinuria (8).

Urine microscopy is particularly helpful in detecting glomerulonephritis and indicating the need for a renal biopsy. Red cell casts and dysmorphic red cells are almost pathognomonic of glomerular bleeding (Table 9). If a fresh sample of urine is microscoped, it is often possible to identify infection quickly, particularly in the presence of a positive nitrite test. Special stains are not usually necessary when examining the urine deposit unless eosinophiluria is suspected (allergic tubulo-interstitial nephritis), or it is necessary precisely to differentiate tubular epithelial cells from pus cells.

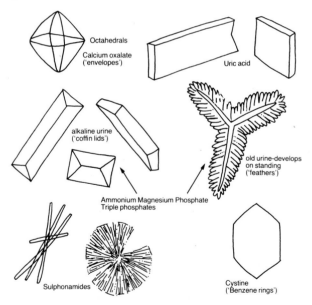

8 **Crystals.** Amorphous deposits of crystals develop with uric acid (acid urine) or with triple phosphates (alkaline urine).

Table 9: Urinary sediment in various disease states

DISEASE	URINE SEDIMENT	
Pre-renal acute renal failure	Minimal abnormality	
Acute tubular necrosis	Granular casts	+++
	Tubular casts	+++
	Tubular cells	+++
	(look for pigment casts if appropriate)	
Nephrotic syndrome	Tubular cells	+
	Leucocytes	+
	Oval fat bodies	++
	Fatty casts	++
	Tubular cell casts	+
Glomerulonephritis (Nephritic syndrome)	Dysmorphic red cells	+++
	Red cell casts	+/+++
	Leucocytes	+
	Tubular cells	+
	(nephrotic features may be present)	
Acute pyelonephritis	Granular casts	++
	Leucocyte casts	+
	Leucocytes	+++
	Tubular cells	++
	Red cells	+
Chronic pyelonephritis	Minimal abnormality	
Cystitis	Leucocytes	++
	Isomorphic red cells	+/++
	Bacteria	++
	No casts	
Chronic renal failure	Minimal abnormality	
	Broad waxy casts	++
	Granular casts	++

Urine cultures

Specimen collection: The urethra usually contains a few bacteria. Micro-organisms multiply rapidly in urine at room temperature. It is therefore essential to collect urine samples for culture correctly as a mid-stream specimen of urine, after cleaning the introitus or penis with sterile water and swabs. The sample must be transported to the laboratory with the minimum of delay or else be stored at 4°C. In infants, a clean catch specimen may suffice but a suprapubic bladder puncture with aspiration of urine may occasionally be necessary. Urine obtained by suprapubic puncture should be sterile. Microscope slides coated with a culture medium may be dipped into the urine stream and then sealed in a sterile bottle and posted to the laboratory for outpatient screening purposes (**9**). If prostatic infection is suspected, split specimens of urine may be cultured. The very first few drops of urine (urethral urine) are placed in one bottle. A conventional mid-stream specimen of urine is then obtained. Following prostatic massage, the next few drops of urine or the expressed prostatic secretion are sent off in separate bottles for culture. A further mid-stream specimen of urine should also be collected and sent for culture.

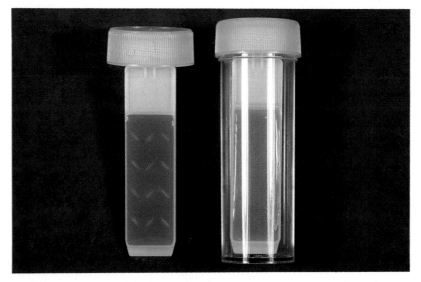

9 Dip slide coated with culture medium (CLED – green: MacConkey – brown) may be used for screening in outpatients (Uricult®).

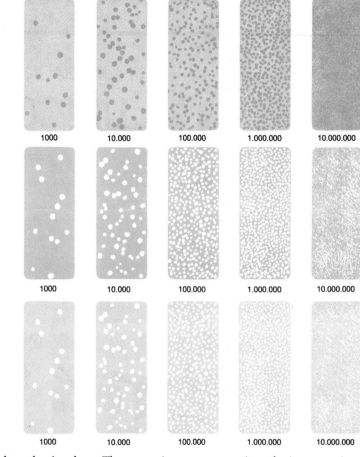

MODEL CHART FOR COLONY DENSITY INDICATING THE NUMBER OF BACTERIA/ml

MacConkey

| 1000 | 10.000 | 100.000 | 1.000.000 | 10.000.000 |

Cled

| 1000 | 10.000 | 100.000 | 1.000.000 | 10.000.000 |

N-Agar

| 1000 | 10.000 | 100.000 | 1.000.000 | 10.000.000 |

10 Colony density chart: The approximate concentration of micro-organisms per millilitre of urine can be gauged from comparison charts such as the one shown (Uricult®). (Reproduced with permission.)

Interpretation of Results

A quantitative count on a properly handled specimen of urine revealing more than 10^5 micro-organisms/ml of urine indicates infection. Lower counts may be indicative of a true infection if urine is very dilute. In general, repeated isolates of the same organism are likely to be due to a true infection. A single organism usually indicates infection, while multiple organisms suggest contamination at the time of collection. Urine without leucocytes is seldom infected.

Urine is usually plated on CLED medium (cystine-lactose electrolyte deficient agar). All the common urinary pathogens grow well on this medium (Table 10). It is electrolyte deficient to prevent the swarming of proteus. The six more important and common bacteria that cause urinary tract infection are shown in **11**, and the main colony characteristics are listed in Table 10.

Special Tests

If tuberculosis is suspected, three early morning urine samples should be set up for TB culture. Occasionally the organism can be identified on Ziehl-Neelsen staining of the urine deposit. In endemic areas, a terminal specimen of urine should be microscoped for the ova of *Schistosoma haematobium*. Certain organisms require special culture media, e.g. viruses, mycoplasma and some fastidious bacteria. If these organisms are suspected, the help of the microbiologist should be enlisted.

Table 10: Colony characteristics of common urinary pathogens on CLED medium

ORGANISM	CLED COLONY CHARACTERISTICS	SIZE (mm)	LACTOSE FERMENTATION
Escherichia coli	yellow	1–2	LF
Klebsiella species	mucoid yellow	1–2	LF
Proteus species	blue	1–2	NLF
Strep. faecalis	yellow	0.5	LF
Pseudomonas aeruginosa	blue usually produce a blue-green pigment	1–2	NLF
Coagulase negative staphs/micrococci	pale white-yellow opaque	0.5	LF
Staph. aureus	yellow-white	0.75	LF
Lactobacilli*	small grey rough surface	0.5	
Coryneforms*	small grey smooth surface	0.5	

LF = Lactose fermenting
NLF = Non-lactose fermenting

*   = **Vaginal flora that may contaminate a mid-stream urine specimen.**

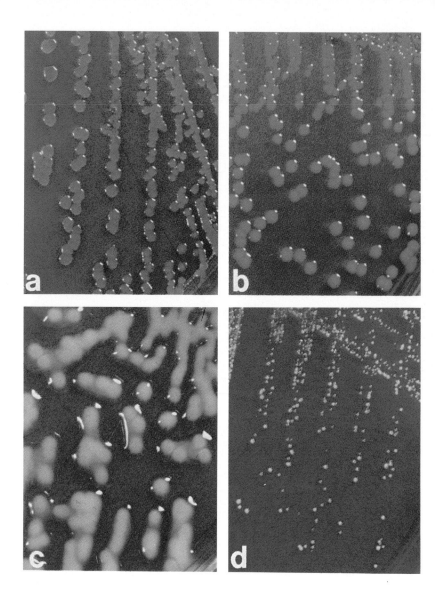

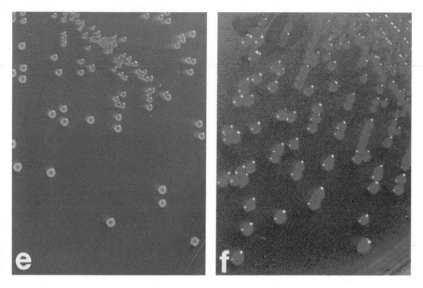

11   Common urinary pathogens: colony characteristics on CLED medium

a. Escherischia coli
b. Proteus mirabilis
c. Klebsiella pneumoniae
d. Micrococcus (Staphyloccocus saprophyticus)
e. Streptococcus faecalis
f. Pseudomonas aeruginosa.

Plasma urea and creatinine

Plasma Urea

Manual techniques: Urea is converted to ammonia and carbon dioxide by the action of urease. A colorimetric method involving either Nessler's reagent or the phenol-hypochlorite reaction of Berthelot is used to measure the ammonia generated.

AutoAnalyzer: The diacetyl-monoxime method of Fearon has been adapted for use in AutoAnalyzer equipment. The urea-containing sample is heated with diacetyl-monoxime, which decomposes to hydroxylamine and diacetyl. Under acidic conditions diacetyl then condenses with urea, giving a coloured product.

Interpretation: The plasma urea concentration reflects the balance between urea production and excretion. As both production and excretion may be influenced by several factors (Table 11), the plasma urea is only a crude guide to renal function. As a single screening test for impaired renal function the plasma creatinine concentration is preferred (see below). Urea production is affected by dietary protein intake, the presence of liver disease and catabolic states, including infection. Urea levels are relatively low in young children and during the recovery phase of acute illnesses (anabolic states). Following a gastro-intestinal haemorrhage, the patient effectively obtains a high protein meal; the plasma urea concentration may rise markedly and disproportionately with respect to changes in plasma creatinine. Urea excretion is also dependent on the urinary flow rate. Once urine excretion falls below 2ml/min. the urea is reclaimed by the tubules by passive back-diffusion. Under conditions of anti-diuresis as much as 70% of the filtered load of urea is reclaimed, whilst during a diuresis the figure falls to 40%.

Plasma Creatinine

Method: True creatinine can be measured by enzymatic degradation using bacterial enzymes. Creatinine has been measured for many years by a method that depends on the production of an orange colour with an alkaline picrate reagent. This method (Jaffé) overestimates creatinine, as other chromogens present in blood (although less so in urine) interfere with the test. True creatinine may also be measured if steps are taken to remove non-creatinine chromogens from the sample (e.g. prior adsorption with Fuller's earth). The current AutoAnalyzer methods involve a dialysis step to exclude both protein some non-creatinine chromogens. Creatinine is then measured by the alkaline picrate method. Some drugs (barbiturates, cephalosporins, ascorbic acid), pyruvic acid and ketones (produced during a diabetic keto-acidosis) may interfere with the measurement of creatinine and can give a falsely elevated value. A high bilirubin concentration leads to a decreased creatinine result. Ingestion of cooked meats causes a post-prandial increase in plasma creatinine.

Table 11: Factors affecting plasma urea and creatinine concentration

RAISED UREA	REDUCED UREA
Impaired GFR	Low protein diet
High protein intake	Starvation
G.I. tract haemorrhage	Liver disease
Catabolic states:	Anabolic states
infection	Polyuria
post-operation	Pregnancy
Reduced urine flow rate	Syndrome of inappropriate ADH
(< 2 ml/min.)	
Dehydration:	
excessive use of diuretics	
Drugs:	
steroids	
most tetracyclines	
RAISED CREATININE	REDUCED CREATININE
Impaired GFR	Small muscle mass
High muscle mass	e.g. elderly
Acute muscle damage	infants
Minimal increase from:	Pregnancy
high meat diet	Syndrome of inappropriate ADH
low urine flow rate	

Interpretation of results: As for urea, the plasma concentration of creatinine reflects the balance between excretion and production. The production of creatinine is largely determined by muscle mass. Thus, the plasma creatinine concentration in children and small adults will be very much lower than that in large, muscular, adult males. The rate of production of creatinine is much more constant than that of urea, but it may be reduced somewhat in advanced renal failure. Creatinine is less affected by diet. With extremely high cooked meat intakes, plasma creatinine may be increased.

Unlike urea excretion, urine flow rate has only a minimal effect on creatinine excretion. Thus, a disproportionate rise in blood urea with respect to blood creatinine can indicate hypovolaemia as well as suggesting an acute gastro-intestinal haemorrhage. Markedly increased liberation of creatinine into the plasma occurs in crush injuries or rhabdomyolysis from any cause.

Despite these reservations, plasma creatinine provides a reliable day-to-day guide to overall renal function, so much so that formulae have been derived to convert a single plasma creatinine concentration into an estimate of (GFR) as indicated by the creatinine clearance:

$$males: \quad Creatinine\ clearance = \frac{100 - 12ml/min/1.73\ m^2}{C}$$

$$females: Creatinine\ clearance = \frac{80 - 7ml/min/1.73\ m^2}{C}$$

$$Where\ C = plasma\ creatinine\ (mg/dl).$$

If serum creatinine values are measured in μmol/l then C in the above formula should be divided by 88.4.

The normal plasma creatinine concentration may be obtained from the following:

$$Plasma\ creatinine\ concentration\ (mg/dl) = 0.004 \times height\ (cm).$$

There is so much reserve renal function that the plasma urea and plasma creatinine do not rise much until the glomerular filtration rate has fallen below 25–30ml/min (**12**).

Once renal function is reduced to less than about 30%, a very steep rise in plasma creatinine occurs for any further change in renal function. It then becomes a very sensitive and accurate measure of further deterioration. To detect changes in renal function between 100% and 30% of normal clearance, techniques are required to measure glomerular filtration rate, as plasma creatinine alone is not sufficiently sensitive.

The exponential rise in plasma creatinine with falling renal function can be demonstrated by plotting the reciprocal or logarithm of the plasma creatinine against time. A straight line may then be obtained which will describe the individual patient's rate of decline to end-stage renal failure. In **13** a hypothetical patient has sustained an acute attack of nephritis, which is controlled but not cured by treatment. Despite cessation of activity in the underlying disease, there is a slow, progressive decline in renal function, which can be plotted as a straight line if the log scale for creatinine is used against time. This simple technique provides a valuable way of following renal function, monitoring the effects of treatment and predicting the time that replacement therapy will be needed. Acute-on-chronic renal failure can be easily recognized if deterioration is more rapid than expected.

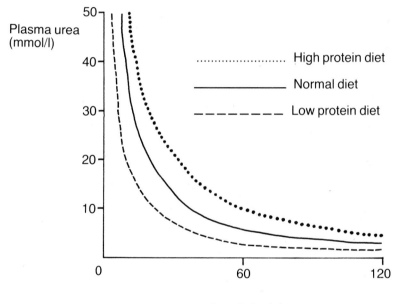

12   Relationship between GFR and plasma urea and the effects of dietary protein

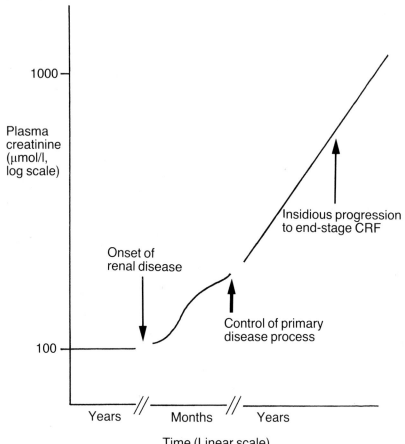

13 Relationship between plasma creatinine and time (semi-log plot). In this graph a hypothetical patient develops renal disease which despite apparent control during the acute or sub-acute phase, eventually progresses to end-stage chronic renal failure.

Plasma electrolytes

Sodium

Measurement: Sodium is measured by flame emission spectrophotometer. Recently, sodium-specific electrodes have been introduced.

Interpretation of results: Sodium is largely extracellular. Sodium regulation is synonymous with regulation of the extracellular fluid volume (ECFV). Disorders of sodium balance will therefore be reflected in changes in ECFV which can be assessed satisfactorily by simple clinical methods (Table 12). Hyper- and hyponatraemia cannot be translated into sodium excess and sodium deficiency respectively as the plasma sodium concentration reflects the ratio of water to sodium and not sodium balance per se. Figures 14 and 15 are based on the classification described by Schrier (see references) and summarise the causes, diagnosis and management of hyper- and hyponatraemia.

Plasma sodium concentration is measured in the water phase of the plasma but is expressed in mmol/l of whole plasma. If there is marked hyperlipidaemia or hyperproteinaemia then the plasma sodium concentration as expressed will be low, so-called 'pseudohyponatraemia'.

Table 12: Assessment of ECFV

EXPANSION	CONTRACTION
Dependent oedema	Reduced tissue turgor
Raised jugular venous pressure	Empty veins
Hypertension	Postural hypotension
Pulmonary congestion	Postural tachycardia
Third heart sound	Poor peripheral perfusion
	Slow capillary filling
CXR: Pulmonary congestion Enlarged heart	CXR: Normal or reduced cardiac silhouette

---

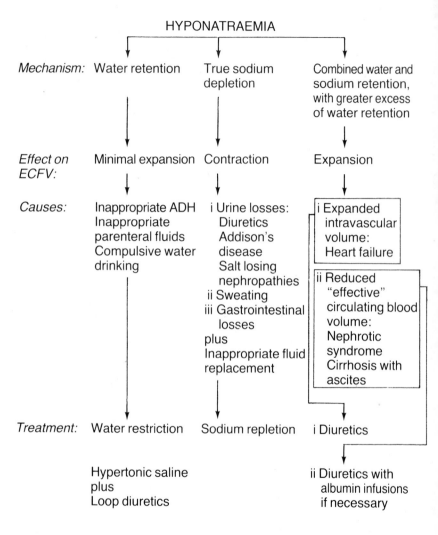

HYPONATRAEMIA

Mechanism:	Water retention	True sodium depletion	Combined water and sodium retention, with greater excess of water retention
Effect on ECFV:	Minimal expansion	Contraction	Expansion
Causes:	Inappropriate ADH Inappropriate parenteral fluids Compulsive water drinking	i Urine losses: Diuretics Addison's disease Salt losing nephropathies ii Sweating iii Gastrointestinal losses plus Inappropriate fluid replacement	i Expanded intravascular volume: Heart failure ii Reduced "effective" circulating blood volume: Nephrotic syndrome Cirrhosis with ascites
Treatment:	Water restriction	Sodium repletion Hypertonic saline plus Loop diuretics	i Diuretics ii Diuretics with albumin infusions if necessary

14   Hyponatraemia

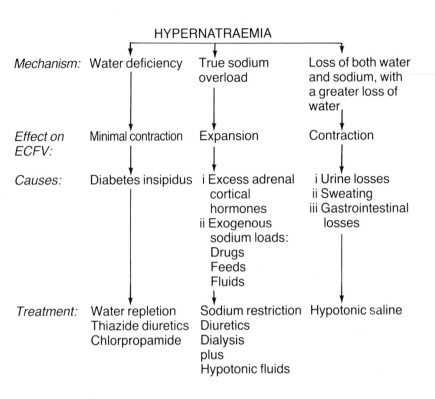

Mechanism:	Water deficiency	True sodium overload	Loss of both water and sodium, with a greater loss of water
Effect on ECFV:	Minimal contraction	Expansion	Contraction
Causes:	Diabetes insipidus	i Excess adrenal cortical hormones ii Exogenous sodium loads: Drugs Feeds Fluids	i Urine losses ii Sweating iii Gastrointestinal losses
Treatment:	Water repletion Thiazide diuretics Chlorpropamide	Sodium restriction Diuretics Dialysis plus Hypotonic fluids	Hypotonic saline

HYPERNATRAEMIA

15 Hypernatraemia

Potassium

Measurement: Potassium can be measured using the same techniques as sodium.

Interpretation of results: Unless there is an additional problem, the plasma potassium concentration remains normal in renal failure so long as urine output is well maintained (i.e. > 1500ml/day). Excessive dietary intake, inappropriately prescribed potassium-conserving diuretics, tissue trauma or oliguria, will lead to alarming and potentially fatal rises in plasma potassium. The common causes of hypo- and hyperkalaemia are

Table 13: Causes of hypo- and hyperkalaemia

HYPOKALAEMIA	HYPERKALAEMIA
Urine losses	Reduced urinary excretion:
1 Secondary to upper G.I. tract chloride loss	Acute/chronic renal failure
2 Diuretics	Type IV RTA
3 Excess adrenocortical hormones	K^+ conserving diuretics
4 Renal tubular acidosis (RTA)	Adrenocortical hormone deficiency
5 Renal artery stenosis (RAS)	Cyclosporin A toxicity
6 Bartter's Syndrome	
7 Liddle's Syndrome	Release from tissues:
8 Ureteric $\rightarrow$ bowel implantation	Rhabdomyolysis
9 Accelerated phase hypertension	Burns
	Haemolysis
	Cytotoxic therapy
Gut losses:	
Diarrhoea	
Upper G.I. tract losses	
Deficient intake	Excess intake
Anabolic states	
Shifts: alkalosis	Shifts: acidosis
Insulin	Hyperkalaemic periodic paralysis
Familial periodic paralysis	

listed in Table 13. In the presence of hypokalaemia, a urinary potassium excretion of more than 20mmol/day suggests a primary renal cause. Prolonged and severe hypokalaemia (e.g. purgative abuse) can produce nephrogenic diabetes insipidus with polyuria, and eventually leads to permanent impairment of renal function with interstitial scarring.

Chloride
Chloride ions form an undissociated soluble salt with mercuric ions. This provides the basis for the mercuric *thiocyanate* AutoAnalyzer method for chloride estimation. Coulometric methods are also widely available for

chloride estimation.

Plasma chloride concentration is helpful in analysing acid-base disturbances. In its grossest form, a profound hypochloraemic metabolic alkalosis follows sustained losses of upper gastro-intestinal secretions. Hypochloraemia is commonly associated with the over-use of diuretics. A hyperchloraemic metabolic acidosis follows hypophosphataemia that may occur with primary hyperparathyroidism.

Bicarbonate

Bicarbonate is measured by assaying the release of carbon dioxide after the addition of acid. In the AutoAnalyzer technique, acid is added and the CO_2 released passes through a silicone membrane and dissolves in an alkaline buffer containing cresol red. The colour change, which is proportional to the pH change, is measured.

Plasma bicarbonate is essential for monitoring acid-base changes, in particular the metabolic acidosis that develops with progressive renal failure. A persistently low plasma bicarbonate in the presence of a urinary pH much above 6 is suggestive of a renal tubular acidosis. A detailed discussion of the assessment of acid-base disturbances is beyond the scope of this book.

Calcium

Measurement of total plasma calcium: Blood samples should be collected in the fasting stage by a venepuncture taken without a tourniquet. Numerous methods are available:

1. EDTA and EGTA titration.
2. Colorimetric methods using creosolphthalein complexone.
3. Fluorometric methods.
4. Atomic absorption spectrometry.

Measurement of ionised plasma calcium: The biologically active form of calcium is the free ionised form. Direct measurement is now possible using a potentiometer with a calcium-sensitive ion-selective electrode. Ionised calcium is of particular value in screening for hyperparathyroidism, and in monitoring vitamin D therapy in renal patients to prevent the development of hypercalcaemia.

Interpretation of results: Forty per cent of total plasma calcium is bound to the plasma proteins, particularly to albumin. The measured total plasma calcium can be corrected for hypoproteinaemia (e.g. nephrotic syndrome) with the following formula:

$$\text{Units: } mg/dl = measured\ calcium - (0.989 \times albumin\ g/dl) + 4$$
$$\text{Units: SI} = measured\ calcium - (0.025 \times albumin\ g/l) + 1$$

Such corrections are not valid with gross disturbances of plasma protein concentration.

Hypercalcaemia per se is nephrotoxic and acute renal failure can develop quite rapidly in the presence of severe hypercalcaemia (e.g. tumour associated). Patients develop polyuria (nephrogenic diabetes insipidus) and dehydration which then further reduces the renal excretion of calcium, exacerbating the hypercalcaemia.

In chronic renal failure, metabolic bone disease may develop due to a combination of 1,25-dihydroxycholecalciferol deficiency, phosphate retention, acidosis and secondary hyperparathyroidism. In most patients there is a moderate depression of the plasma calcium. Should a patient with chronic renal failure have a normal or elevated plasma calcium, then the patient should be screened for an underlying multiple myeloma, primary hyperparathyroidism and aluminium intoxication. Later in the natural history of renal bone disease, autonomous tertiary hyperparathyroidism (hypercalcaemic hyperparathyroidism) may develop. The patient becomes hypercalcaemic even though Vitamin D and calcium supplements have been withdrawn. Parathyroidectomy is then required.

Patients with rhabdomyolysis and acute renal failure may have profound hypocalcaemia at presentation as the damaged muscles bind calcium. Later, during the recovery phase, marked hypercalcaemia may be seen. This is due to various factors including the release of bound calcium from damaged muscles, persisting secondary hyperparathyroidism and the restoration of 1,25-dihydroxycholecalciferol synthesis by the recovering kidneys.

Patients with the nephrotic syndrome lose considerable amounts of Vitamin D binding protein with their proteinuria, and may develop 25–OHD_3 deficiency. As already noted above, the measured plasma total calcium concentration in these patients will be low as the result of hypoproteinaemia.

Phosphate

The method of Fiske and Subbarow is generally used. An acid solution of ammonium molybdate is reacted with phosphate to form ammonium phosphomolybdate. The product is reduced under controlled conditions to produce molybdenum blue in amounts proportional to the concentration of phosphate present.

Phosphate retention is found in acute and chronic renal failure. An elevated plasma phosphate depresses the plasma ionised calcium concentration, producing secondary hyperparathyroidism and metastatic calcification. Plasma phosphate can be controlled by aluminium hydroxide given with food. Excessive treatment leads to phosphate depletion and osteomalacia. In the tumour lysis syndrome the plasma phosphate concentration can rise dramatically and may be one of the factors responsible for acute renal failure in this syndrome. A variety of renal tubular disorders (proximal tubule) may be associated with an inappropriate leak of phosphate in the urine. Phosphaturia is also a feature of hyperparathyroidism in the presence of normal renal function. Hypophosphataemia may also develop in renal transplant patients in the absence of hyperparathyroidism due to increased sensitivity of the renal tubule to PTH.

Anion Gap

The anion gap is defined as:

$$(Na^+ + K^+) - (Cl^- + HCO_3^-)$$
$$Normal\ range:\ 6{-}16mmol/l.$$

Thus, the anion gap, although estimated from the concentration of sodium, potassium, chloride and bicarbonate, is actually determined by the concentration of unmeasured anions and cations.

Unmeasured cations		*Unmeasured anions*	
Calcium	= 2.5	*Protein*	= 15.0
Magnesium	= 1.0	*Phosphate*	= 1.0
Total:	**3.5 mmol/l**	*Sulphate*	= 0.5
		Organic acids	= 3.0
		Total:	**19.5 mmol/l**

19.5–3.5 = 16
Anion gap = 16.

The term 'anion gap' is a misnomer because it implies that there is a gap between anions and cations. In fact, the laws of electrochemical neutrality require that the total cations should be balanced by an equal number of anions.

An increased anion gap implies the presence of another anion such as one of the organic acids that accumulate in renal failure or in diabetic keto-acidosis (Table 14).

Table 14: Anion gap

HIGH ANION GAP	LOW ANION GAP
Metabolic acidosis:	Dilution
Impaired removal:	Hypoalbuminaemia
Renal failure	Bromism
Dehydration	
Increased production:	Excess cations:
Diabetic keto-acidosis	Paraproteins
Starvation	Hypercalcaemia
Lactic acidosis	Hypermagnesaemia
Alcoholic keto-acidosis	Lithium toxicity
Inborn errors of metabolism	
Ingestion:	
Salicylate	
Paraldehyde	
Methanol	
Ethylene Glycol	

3: INTERMEDIATE INVESTIGATIONS

Ultrasound

Ultrasound is a quick, cheap and non-invasive technique for imaging the kidneys. It has a role to play in the early screening investigations of the patient with suspected renal disease. In skilled hands, with modern techniques, several important diagnostic questions may be answered. In the initial assessment of the patient with suspected renal disease, we need to know whether or not the patient actually has two kidneys. If so, we also need to know whether they are of normal size and shape and if they are non-obstructed (16). Dilatation typical of obstruction is easily demonstrable by ultrasound (17). Ultrasound can answer many different questions accurately and quickly (Table 15).

Inflammation of the kidneys makes them more echogenic, so that the inflamed renal parenchyma appears brighter than the liver on ultrasound scanning. Space-occupying lesions can be grouped into those that are solid (malignant until proved otherwise) or cystic (19). The technique can be used for screening families for polycystic kidneys (21). Extrarenal collections (22) and masses pressing on the kidney or ureter (23) can also be demonstrated. The ultrasound may also distinguish between acute and chronic obstruction, as in chronic obstruction there is very little identifiable cortical thickness. This finding usually implies a disappointing result from the surgical relief of obstruction (18).

Plain X-ray of the kidney, ureter and bladder areas (KUB)

A plain X-ray of the entire urinary tract is taken prior to any further specialised X-rays (24 and 25). Even if an IVU is not going to be carried out, it may be wise to have a plain X-ray as this is the best way of detecting any calcification in the renal tract (26). Sometimes the plain abdominal film will demonstrate the kidney outlines quite clearly, particularly if there is much peri-renal fat. Most urinary tract calculi are radio-opaque, so that if the renal areas and outlines of ureter and bladder are carefully scrutinised calculi may be spotted (24 and 28). An IVU will be necessary to confirm that the calcification noted on a plain X-ray film does, in fact, lie within the renal tract. Oblique and lateral films may be needed to prove this. Occasionally gas may be noted in the renal tract when gas-producing organisms cause a urinary tract infection, as may happen in diabetes mellitus (27).

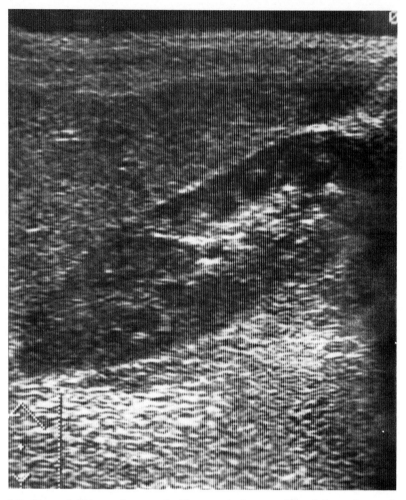

16 Normal kidney ultrasound: The cortex is smooth and free of complex echoes. The renal pyramids are clearly shown and there is no dilatation of the renal pelvis or calyces.

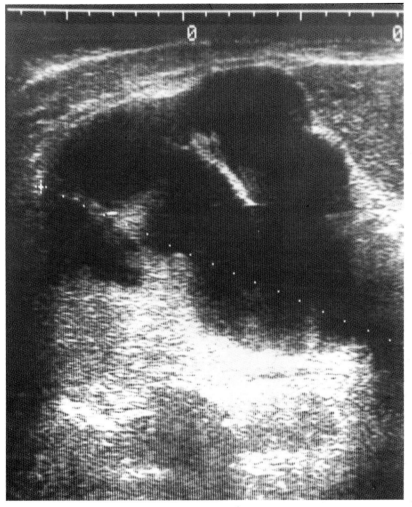

17 Ultrasound: chronic obstruction. Gross dilatation of the renal pelvis and calyces with thinning of the overlying cortex can be seen.

Table 15: The role of ultrasound in the investigation of kidney disease

1   Presence or absence of kidneys

2   Kidney mass:
       Size and shape of kidneys
       Cortical thickness

3   Obstruction:
       Presence or absence of dilatation of
       calyces and renal pelvis

4   Space-occupying lesions:
       Solid
       Cystic

5   Calcification:
       Parenchymal
       Within the collecting system and pelvis

6   Parenchymal inflammation

7   Peri-renal collections

8   Bladder:
       Residual urine volume after micturition

9   Control of invasive procedures:
       Renal biopsy
       Cyst aspiration
       Percutaneous pyelogram and nephrostomy

10 Early detection of renal transplant rejection

11 Patency of inferior vena cava and renal veins

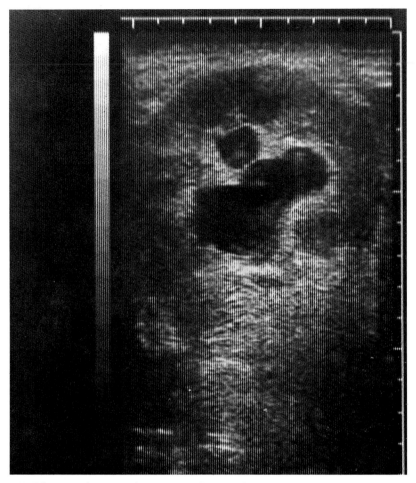

18 Ultrasound: acute obstruction. There is dilatation of the renal pelvis and calyces but there is preservation of a good thickness of surrounding cortex.

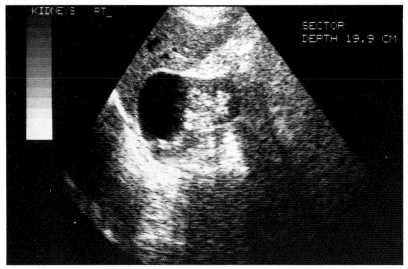

19 Ultrasound: simple cyst. The large cyst to the left of the renal shadow has no echoes within it and represents a simple (benign) cyst.

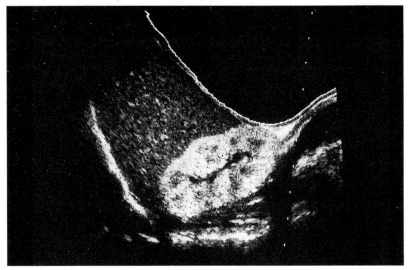

20 Ultrasound: congenital oxalosis. Note the very bright (echogenic) kidney of congenital oxalosis due to the early deposition of oxalate crystals not yet visible on a plain abdominal X-ray, in an infant aged two months.

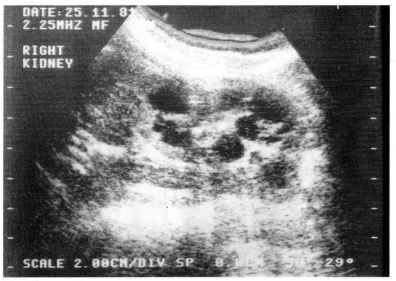

21 Ultrasound: congenital polycystic kidneys. The multiple parenchymal cysts of congenital polycystic kidneys are clearly shown.

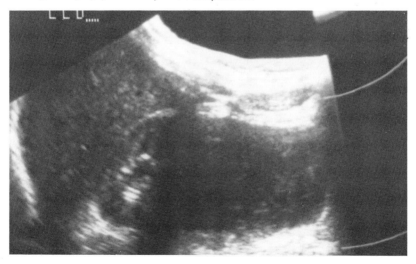

22 Ultrasound: perirenal haematoma. Rupture of the kidney with the formation of a large haematoma can be seen to the right of the renal outline in a patient who sustained a road traffic accident.

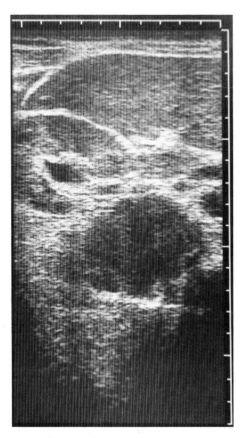

23 Ultrasound: extrarenal obstruction. The kidney demonstrates obstruction with dilatation of the renal pelvis which has been caused by a mass of neoplastic glands compressing the ureter.

Intravenous urogram (IVU)

Method

Patients should be prepared for an IVU with an aperient to reduce bowel and gas shadows that may obscure details of the renal tract. Dehydration was traditionally requested (e.g. nil by mouth for 4–8 hours) to enhance concentration of the urine. This is contraindicated in the presence of renal impairment as contrast nephrotoxicity may be increased in the dehydrated subject. In renal impairment large doses of the newer non-ionic contrast media should be given. For the IVU an intravenous injection of radio-opaque contrast material is given. The agent chosen is excreted by the kidney by glomerular filtration only. X-rays are taken before injection and at precise intervals thereafter to demonstrate contrast within the kidney substance (nephrogram), the collecting system (pyelogram) and ureter and bladder (29, 30). The film taken immediately after the end of the contrast injection provides information about perfusion of the kidneys and is the baseline from which to assess the time course of the nephrogram. Further films are taken after micturition to assess bladder emptying. Late films (12 and 24 hours) may be necessary in patients in whom obstruction is suspected (32 and 33).

Dose
If renal failure is present, then a high dose of contrast must be used. Prior dehydration is not necessary and can seriously damage renal function in the patient with pre-existing renal impairment. The newer non-ionic contrast agents are to be preferred.

Risks
There is a small risk of an allergic reaction to the contrast media. Patients with diabetes mellitus may develop acute renal failure after an IVU, as

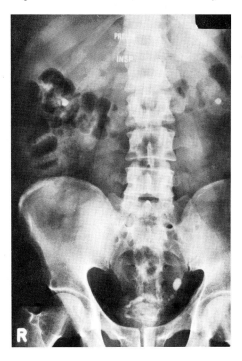

24 KUB: plain X-ray taken as a preliminary to a formal IVU. Note the multiple areas of calcification which appear to overlie both kidneys, the lower left ureter and the bladder area. The pelvic calcification is within the wall of the bladder and is typical of that induced by schistosomiasis. The resulting bladder fibrosis produces vesico-ureteric obstruction and favours the development of upper tract infection and calculi (see 34).

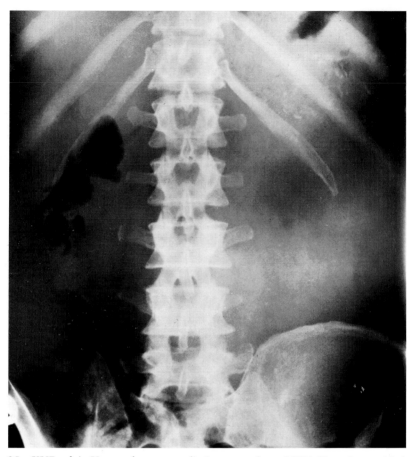

25 KUB: plain X-ray taken as a preliminary to a formal IVU. Note the speckled calcification related to the lower ribs on the left. This sort of calcification is typical of a renal tumour. Note also the suggestion of a mass displacing bowel gas shadows to the patient's right.

the contrast appears to be particularly nephrotoxic in this group of patients. Jaundice also accentuates the nephrotoxic potential of X-ray contrast material. In multiple myeloma the contrast, if combined with prior dehydration, may lead to acute renal failure from tubular obstruction. The volume of contrast constitutes a significant osmotic and sodium load and can precipitate heart failure in susceptible patients.

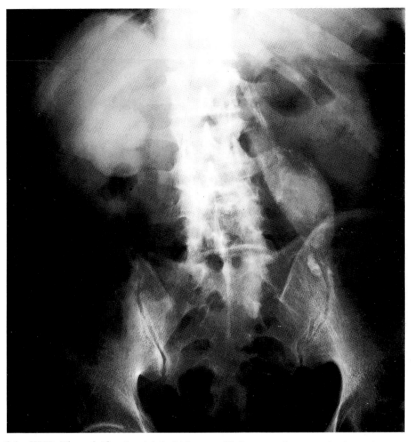

26 KUB: The calcification (right kidney and left psoas abscess) of tuberculosis is shown in addition to a small opacity in the left pelvis (ureteric stone).

Interpretation of Results

The sequence of events that occurs in the normal kidney after the injection of radiographic contrast is demonstrated in **29**. A one-minute film taken immediately after the end of the contrast injection is a measure of renal perfusion, and indicates size and shape. On later films details of calyces are shown. For ease of interpretation, abnormal IVU's are best

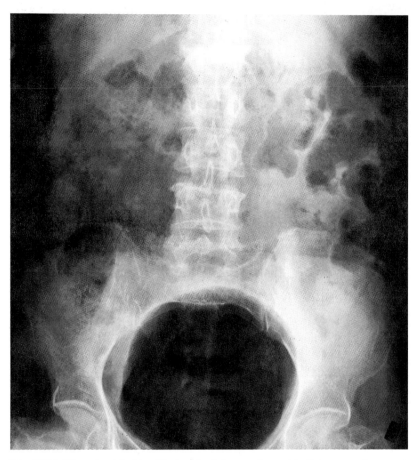

27   KUB: There is a bladder filled with air in a patient with diabetes mellitus and a urinary tract infection with gas producing micro-organisms.

divided into those with normal and those with abnormal calyces, and also on the basis of kidney size (Tables 16 and 17). In the presence of obstruction the passage of contrast through the kidney is delayed, occurring gradually as sodium and water are progressively reabsorbed from the nephron. This gives the characteristic features of obstruction which include a slowly developing and delayed nephrogram, with the subsequent late demonstration of a dilated collecting system (**32–34**).

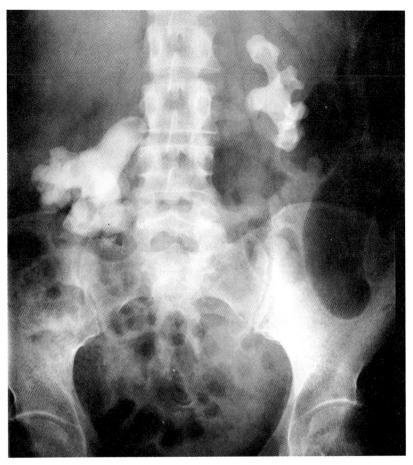

28 KUB: Large bilateral staghorn calculi are clearly visible. Note that X-ray contrast media has not yet been given and that the calculi almost completely fill the renal pelvis and calyces on both sides.

Sometimes obstruction is so gross that the calyces never fill. They may then be outlined by contrast within the kidney substance and appear as a negative pyelogram. In acute tubular necrosis there appears to be recirculation of contrast with little excretion. An immediate dense and persistent nephrogram develops, which lasts until the contrast has been excreted in the bile (**31**).

Table 16: Abnormal IVU

CALYCEAL PATTERN

Normal calyces	*Abnormal calyces*

Glomerulonephritis	Displacement:
	  Cyst(s)
	  Tumours

Interstitial nephritis	

Hypertension and renal artery stenosis	Destruction:
	  Papillary necrosis
	  Tuberculosis
	  Chronic pyelonephritis

Diabetes mellitus (unless papillary necrosis)	

Amyloidosis	Dilatation:
	  Obstruction
	  Reflux

Infarcts	
Ischaemia	Medullary sponge kidney
Foetal lobulation	Medullary cystic disease
Compensatory hypertrophy	Congenital abnormalities and variations
Hypoplastic kidneys	Previous surgery

Table 17: Kidney size

Small	*Large*
Most chronic renal disease	Polycystic kidneys
Renal artery stenosis (ipsilateral)	Compensatory hypertrophy
Congenital hypoplasia	Diabetes mellitus (even if CRF)
	Amyloidosis (even if CRF)
	Most acute renal disease
	Renal vein thrombosis
	Obstruction
	Infiltration (e.g. leukaemia)
	Tumours

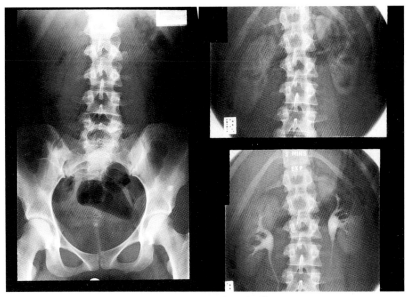

29 (A) **Normal IVU.** Preliminary KUB and early films.

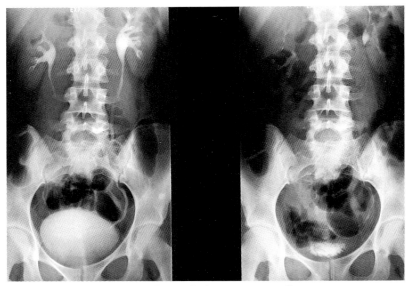

29 (B) **Normal IVU.** Later film and after micturition film.

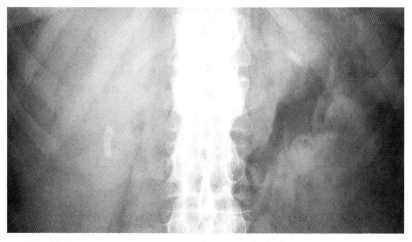

30 (A) Plain X-ray prior to contrast showing calcified opacities (papillae) over both renal outlines.

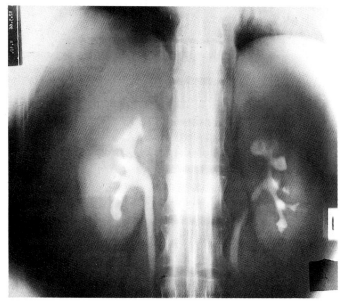

30 (B) Post contrast film showing calyceal distortions (ring shadow, horns, egg-in-cup) typical of analgesic nephropathy.

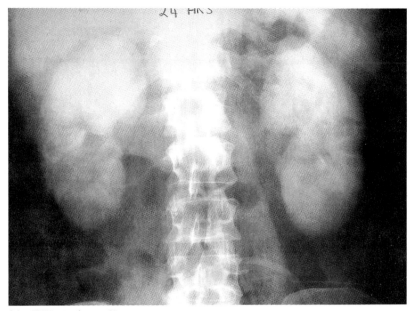

31 IVU: 24-hour film (IVU) demonstrating the persistent dense nephrogram typical of acute tubular necrosis (ATN). Note the lack of pyelogram.

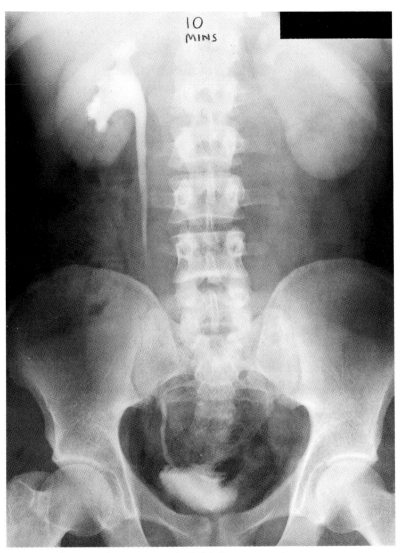

32 IVU showing obstruction to the left kidney. Note the well established pyelogram and ureterogram on the normal right side. Excretion on the left is markedly delayed with only a nephrogram demonstrable at ten minutes (see 33).

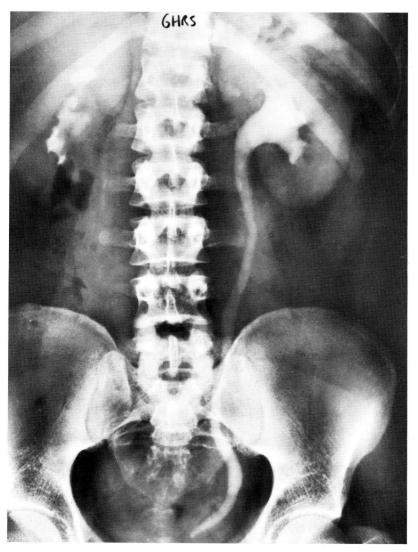

33 **IVU delayed films of the same patient as in 32.** Note the normal right side from which contrast has nearly completely drained. By comparison, the left side shows a moderately dilated renal pelvis with ballooned calyces and a dilated ureter. The obstruction can be seen to be at the level of the vesico-ureteric junction where a small stone was subsequently demonstrated.

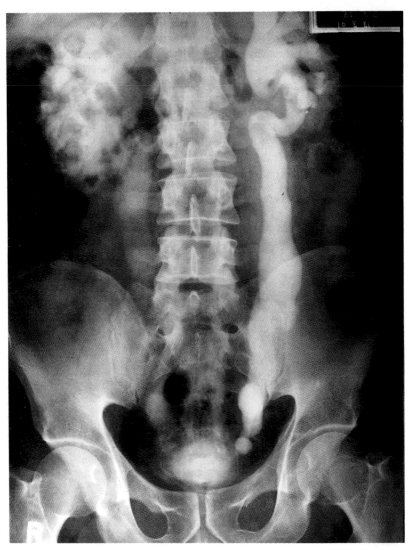

34 Late after micturition (AM) film from an IVU series of the same patient as shown in 24. Bladder wall calcification is partly obscured by the contrast but gross bilateral ureteric dilatation and bilateral hydronephrosis from vesico-ureteric obstruction are shown. Bladder carcinoma may develop as a late complication of schistosomiasis. Stones, as shown in **24**, are a complication of stasis plus infection.

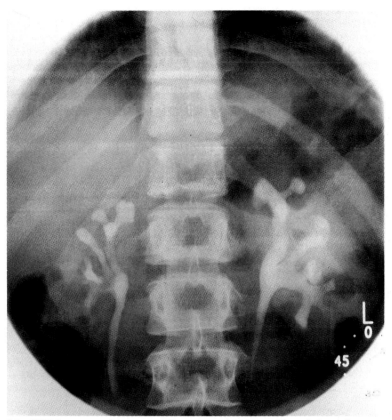

35   IVU demonstrating two small contracted kidneys. There is loss of cortex and clubbing with distortion of the calyces. These are the features of chronic (reflux) pyelonephritis (reflux nephropathy). New cortical scars rarely develop after the age of five years in the absence of obstruction.

Clearance techniques

The concept of clearance
Clearance is a theoretical concept. It measures the volume of plasma containing the amount of any given substance that is actually excreted by the kidney in a unit of time. It is measured in ml/min.

$$The\ amount\ removed = \frac{Urine\ volume \times Urine\ concentration}{Time}$$

$$The\ volume\ of\ plasma\ cleared = \frac{U \times V}{T \times P}\ ml/min.$$

$U = Urine\ concentration$
$V = Urine\ volume/24\ hours$
$T = Time\ (1440\ mins/24\ hours)$
$P = Plasma\ concentration$

Two valuable indices of renal function can be obtained using clearance values (**36** and Table 18).

a) *The clearance of a substance freely filtered at the glomerulus and not secreted or reabsorbed by the tubules will measure glomerular filtration rate (GFR).*
b) *The clearance of a substance that is both filtered and secreted by the tubules so as to be completely cleared from the plasma in one passage through the kidney will measure renal plasma flow (RPF).*

Estimation of glomerular filtration rate (GFR)
The best overall single index of renal function is the glomerular filtration rate. With progressive renal disease and scarring it is thought that nephrons drop out progressively, whether the original disease is primarily glomerular or tubular-interstitial. GFR is a measure of the functional capacity of the remaining nephrons.

Inulin clearance: To measure GFR there needs to be a substance in the blood that is filtered at the glomerulus as freely as water, but is neither secreted nor reabsorbed by the tubules (Table 18). No naturally occurring substance meets these requirements. For many years physiologists have used Inulin (a fructose polymer, M.W. 5,000), given by continuous intravenous infusions over several hours to produce steady state conditions with a stable plasma concentration.

Filtered load of Inulin = GFR × Plasma concentration of Inulin
Amount of Inulin excreted = Urine volume × Urine concentration of Inulin

For Inulin or for a similar ideal substance these two will be the same during the steady state.

$$GFR \times Plasma\ concentration = Urine\ volume \times Urine\ concentration\ of\ Inulin$$

$$GFR = \frac{UV}{P \times T}\ ml/min$$

where U = Urine concentration
V = Urine volume (24 hours)
P = Plasma concentration
T = 1440 (minutes/24 hours).

AutoAnalyzer techniques for the measurement of Inulin have been devised and isotopically labelled Inulin is now available.

Accurate urine collection really requires a urethral catheter, which is clearly unsuitable for routine clinical use. It is, however, possible to calculate clearance without the need for urine collection as follows:

Given that Inulin clearance $= \dfrac{UI \times V}{PI}$ *ml/min, then, during the steady*

state phase of an intravenous infusion of Inulin the infusion rate (Inf) will be the same as the excretion rate (UI × V).

$$Thus\ clearance = \frac{Inf}{PI}$$

where UI = Urine concentration of Inulin (mg/ml)
PI = Plasma concentration of Inulin (mg/ml)
V = Urine flow rate (ml/min), and
Inf = Infusion rate of Inulin (mg/min).

Method: Approximately 35mg/kg body weight of Inulin is given as an intravenous bolus. Thereafter Inulin is infused at a rate of 0.1mg/kg body weight/min. A steady state is usually reached by 60 minutes, at which time the plasma concentration of Inulin is taken every 15 minutes for a further hour. The concentration of Inulin in the infusion fluid and the infusion rate must be accurately measured. Then, as shown above, the GFR under steady state conditions is obtained from

$$\frac{Infusion\ rate\ (mg/min)}{Plasma\ Inulin\ concentration\ (mg/ml)}$$

Inulin dose should be reduced in renal failure.

Creatinine clearance: Endogenous creatinine is freely filtered at the glomerulus, but some creatinine is also secreted by the tubules. Plasma creatinine remains fairly constant in a given individual with stable renal function. Endogenous creatinine clearance is widely used as the clinician's measurement of GFR. As renal function fails, the proportion of excreted creatinine that is secreted by the tubules falls, so that creatinine clearance more accurately reflects GFR (37). In patients with the nephrotic syndrome, there may be a marked increase in the amount of creatinine secreted by the tubules, such that the creatinine clearance may grossly over-estimate GFR. By comparison, urea is also freely filtered at the glomerulus but diffuses from the tubules and is reabsorbed during its passage along the nephron. Back-diffusion is particularly important under conditions of low urine flow rate. Therefore, urea clearance under-estimates GFR, but as renal failure develops the proportion of urea that is reabsorbed falls (37) as hyperperfusion of the remaining nephrons occurs.

The mean of creatinine clearance and urea clearance is therefore a more accurate measure of GFR than either alone (37).

The method of measuring creatinine clearance as outlined above has traditionally relied on the collection of a 24-hour urine sample. It is surprisingly difficult to obtain a complete and accurate 24-hour urine collection. One way around this problem is to measure the creatinine clearance on two consecutive days and, if the figures do not agree, then the measurements must be repeated. Another technique is to carry out two closely timed and well supervised two- or four-hour urine collections, calculating creatinine clearance from values for plasma creatinine taken in the middle of each collection period. Perhaps the most accurate way of performing a creatinine clearance is to collect overnight urine only. The patient is asked to void completely on retiring (as most do anyway) and again on rising. This urine, and any passed during the night is all that is used. The time of retiring and rising are noted.

Variation in the daily intake of cooked meat is likely to influence both the plasma concentration and urinary excretion of creatinine. When no proper attention is paid to diet and urine flow rate, creatinine clearance values may vary, since the plasma creatinine concentration is measured in the morning when the concentration is lowest. Creatinine clearance may underestimate GFR when urine flow rate is below 0.5ml/minute.

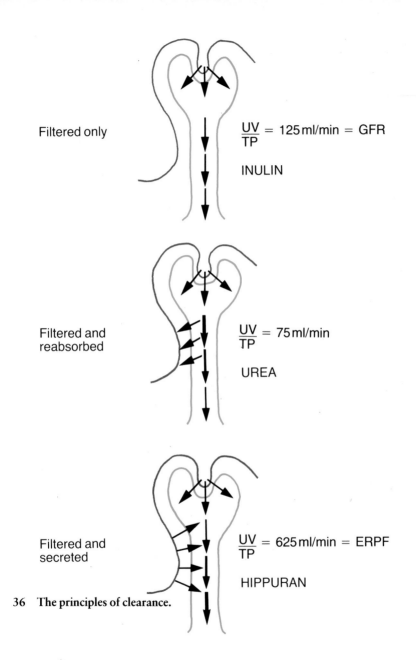

Filtered only $\dfrac{UV}{TP} = 125\,ml/min = GFR$

INULIN

Filtered and reabsorbed $\dfrac{UV}{TP} = 75\,ml/min$

UREA

Filtered and secreted $\dfrac{UV}{TP} = 625\,ml/min = ERPF$

HIPPURAN

36 The principles of clearance.

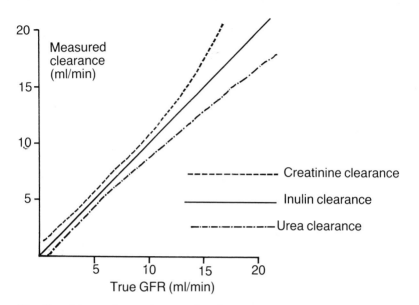

37 Creatinine and urea clearance in relation to inulin clearance

Table 18: Clearance studies

SUBSTANCE	MEASUREMENT	NORMAL VALUES (ml/min) (Corrected for 1.73 m² body surface area)
Inulin B_{12} (^{57}Co or ^{58}Co) EDTA (^{51}Cr) }	GFR	MALES 100–150 FEMALES 95–125
Creatinine	Approximate GFR (over-estimates)	MALES 110–160 FEMALES 100–130
Urea	Approximate GFR (under-estimates)	55–75
Para-amino-hippuric acid (PAH) Orthohippuric acid (^{125}I Hippuran) }	ERPF	MALES 500–700 FEMALES 450–650

Isotopic measurement of GFR: Methods that do not rely on urine collection have been devised using the disappearance rate of isotopically labelled agents from the blood. Vitamin B_{12}, EDTA and DTPA are small molecular weight substances that can be given intravenously. They are freely filtered and not handled by the tubules to any significant extent. They all give a good estimate of true GFR. ^{51}Cr EDTA is the agent now most widely used.

1. A baseline blood sample is taken to ensure no residual radio-activity from any previous investigations.
2. An accurately measured amount of ^{51}Cr EDTA ($50\,\mu Ci$) is given by careful intravenous injection. This is best done through a butterfly cannula and then washed into the vein with 5ml of normal saline. The precise time of injection is noted. (The syringe that contained the labelled EDTA is returned to the laboratory.)
3. Four precisely timed blood samples are taken from the arm *not* used for the injection. Timing depends on the degree of renal impairment expected:

Blood samples	Normal or moderately impaired	Grossly impaired
Baseline	*Pre-injection*	*Pre-injection*
2nd	2hr	2hr
3rd	3hr	6hr
4th	4hr	12hr
5th	5hr	18hr

GFR can be estimated from the slope of the disappearance of the injected ^{51}Cr EDTA. No urine samples are needed.

The mathematical principle used to calculate GFR makes several assumptions which are not entirely true, i.e. GFR is assumed to remain constant over the test period and there is assumed to be a rapid and even distribution of the ^{51}Cr EDTA.

For comparison between different patients, GFR and plasma creatinine should be corrected for body surface area ($1.73m^2$). This is particularly important for children. Nomograms are widely available for this purpose (see appendix). Body surface area may also be calculated from the following:

$$Log\ A = (0.425\ log\ W) + (0.725\ log\ H) + 1.8564$$
$$where\ A = Body\ surface\ area\ (cm^2)$$
$$W = Weight\ (kg)$$
$$H = Height\ (cm)$$

(To convert inches to centimetres multiply by 2.54.
To convert pounds to kilograms multiply by 0.454).

Effective renal plasma flow (ERPF)

As already discussed, the clearance of a substance that is completely removed from the plasma by glomerular filtration, followed by tubular secretion, will measure renal plasma flow. For many years para-amino-hippuric acid (PAH) has been used. The concentration in the plasma of the test substance must not be sufficient to saturate the tubular secretory mechanisms (e.g. plasma PAH < 5mg/dl). PAH is only 90% extracted by the kidneys, so it under-estimates renal blood flow. Presumably, some of the blood reaching the kidney does not go to functioning glomeruli and nephrons. For this reason, PAH clearance is said to measure effective renal plasma flow (ERPF). PAH cannot be isotopically labelled and its chemical estimation is difficult. Orthohippuric acid (Hippuran) can be readily labelled with iodine and may be used instead. [123]I has a short half-life and is therefore too expensive for routine use. [125]I has a longer 'shelf-life' and lower energy radiation and is to be preferred to ^{131}I for routine use. It is difficult to obtain iodinated orthohippuric acid pure so that some iodine will be free. It therefore underestimates true renal plasma flow but, nevertheless, is of value.

One-shot method

1. A baseline blood sample (10ml heparin tube) should be taken to exclude any pre-existing radio-activity from previous investigations.
2. An accurate injection of a defined amount of [125]I Hippuran ($50\,\mu$Ci) is given via a butterfly needle and washed into the vein with 5ml of sterile normal saline. The syringe may be returned to the Isotope Laboratory for weighing or counting. The time of injection must be noted.
3. Timed blood samples are taken every five minutes for 45 minutes following injection. Samples should be taken from the *opposite* arm from that used to inject the [125]I Hippuran. ERPF can be calculated from the disappearance curve.

Measurement of ERPF is seldom used in routine clinical practice, but is still of value for detailed studies in clinical research. ERPF measurement using [125]I Hippuran can be combined with GFR measurements using ^{51}Cr EDTA at the same sitting. A further index of renal function, the filtration fraction, can be calculated.

$$Filtration\ fraction = \frac{GFR}{ERPF} = 0.2$$

ERPF – Normal values (corrected for 1.73m² body surface area):
Males: 654 ± 163ml/min.
Females: 592 ± 153ml/min.

Infusion method: As with the measurement of the clearance of Inulin, PAH clearance (CPAH) can be measured without the need for urine collection during an infusion, once a steady state has been reached. The infusion rate depends upon the renal function and is estimated from the patient's creatinine clearance measured just prior to the test.

The desired plasma level of PAH is approximately 2mg/dl. Thus:

$$CPAH = \frac{UPAH \times V}{PPAH}\ ml/min.$$

If one assumes a normal filtration fraction –

$$CPAH = 5 \times Creatinine\ clearance$$

To maintain a steady state at a plasma concentration of 2mg/dl, the

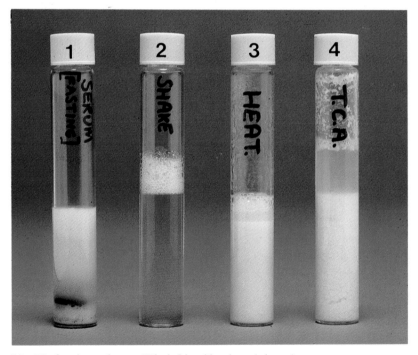

38 Nephrotic syndrome: Whole blood has been left to clot at room temperature revealing markedly lipaemic serum (1). If urine is shaken it froths and the froth persists due to proteinuria (2). When urine is heated (3) or if trichloroacetic acid (TCA) is added (4) a heavy precipitate of protein develops.

infusion rate should equal the excretion rate. Thus:

Infusion rate (mg/min) = 5 × Creatinine clearance × 0.02.

A loading dose of about 10mg/kg body weight of PAH is given. If renal function is nearly normal, then the infusion rate will be about 0.4mg/kg body weight per minute. A steady state is reached after about 60 minutes, at which time blood is taken every 15 minutes to check that a steady state has indeed been reached. The concentration of PAH in the infusion fluid is checked and the rate of infusion accurately measured.

$$ERPF = \frac{Excretion\ of\ PAH}{PPAH}$$

Excretion of PAH (mg/min) = Infusion of PAH (mg/min)

Therefore:

$$ERPF = \frac{Infusion\ rate\ of\ PAH}{PPAH}$$

where PPAH is the steady state plasma concentration of PAH. When renal function is markedly impaired, a longer time period is required to reach the steady state.

Proteinuria

Causes
Normal urine contains less than 250mg of protein per 24 hours. When present, proteinuria may arise in one of the following ways:

1. Glomerular leak of normal plasma proteins (albumin, immunoglobulins, etc.).
2. Overflow of proteins that are present in the blood in abnormally high concentration (light chains, haemoglobin, myoglobin).
3. Tubular damage and impaired reabsorption of low molecular weight proteins (β_2 microglobulin).
4. Tubular secretion (Tamm-Horsfall protein – normally $\leq$ 100mg/24hrs).
5. Release of damaged cells and debris into the renal tract.
6. Chyluria.

Screening tests
The use of stick tests has already been described. They are so sensitive (300mg/l) that a positive test does not necessarily mean that there is significant disease, particularly if the urine volume is only 500ml/24 hours. It is also important to remember that significant renal diseases can

occur in the absence of proteinuria. A positive stick test must be confirmed by one of the quantitative tests. Other nonspecific screening tests are shown in (**38**).

Confirmation and quantitation

Sulphosalicylic acid (Turbidimetric method): A positive stick test for proteinuria may be confirmed by adding 10 drops (0.5ml) of a 25% solution of sulphosalicylic acid to 5ml of urine to produce precipitation. This test will detect approximately 200mg protein/l of urine. False positives may occur with penicillin, radiographic contrast media, sulphonamides and tolbutamide.

Biuret method: A formal 24-hour urine collection should be made and the protein precipitated with trichloroacetic acid. The precipitate is assayed for protein using the biuret test. Concentrations of protein above 50mg protein/l can be detected by this method.

In order to use serial estimations of proteinuria as a guide to the severity of glomerular lesions, and to follow the responses to treatment, two points should be borne in mind. If plasma protein concentration falls markedly, then the total 24-hour urine protein excretion will also fall. Secondly, if GFR falls, then proteinuria may also fall as the number of functioning nephrons drops. Measurement of an albumin clearance or expression of proteinuria as a ratio with creatinine excretion overcomes these two problems.

Types of proteinuria: The most specific way of defining the type of proteinuria (glomerular or tubular) is to carry out polyacrylamide gel or cellulose acetate electrophoresis on the urine specimen (**39** and **40**). A pattern similar to that of plasma with high molecular weight proteins present suggests a non-selective or glomerular type of proteinuria. The absence of high molecular weight immunoglobulins and the presence of predominantly low molecular weight proteins such as β_2 microglobulin indicate that tubular damage and failure of reabsorption is responsible for the proteinuria (Table 19). β_2 microglobulin is freely filtered at the glomerulus, but almost completely reabsorbed by the proximal tubule under normal conditions. Up to $370\mu g$ of β_2 microglobulin passes to the urine daily. The ratio of urine β_2 microglobulins to albumin in the urine separates tubular from glomerular proteinuria. Excessive production of free light chains is followed by their appearance in the urine as Bence-Jones protein. The classical heating test for Bence-Jones protein, in which the precipitation of protein occurs at 60°C, followed by resolution on boiling, has now been replaced by immuno-electrophoresis of the urine. This technique not only demonstrates the presence of light chains in the urine, but also identifies whether or not they are all of the same type (monoclonal kappa or lambda light chains).

In general, glomerular proteinuria is usually above 2–3g/24 hours, while tubular proteinuria is normally less than 2g/24 hours. Proteinuria in excess of 3g/24 hours/m² body surface area is defined as nephrotic being associated with oedema, hypoproteinaemia and hyperlipidaemia.

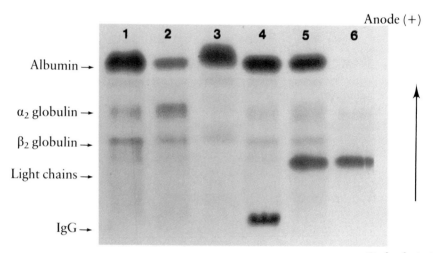

1. Normal serum
2. Nephrotic syndrome – serum
3. Nephrotic syndrome – urine (concentrated ×10)
4. IgG myeloma – serum
5. Bence-Jones only myeloma – serum
6. Bence-Jones only myeloma – urine (concentrated ×50)

39 Electrophoresis of concentrated urine and serum on cellulose acetate (250 volts, 5mAmps, 20 minutes). Nephrotic serum has a reduced albumin, reduced globulin and increased α_2 globulin. The serum of the patient with multiple myeloma has a distinct monoclonal band (M-band). In the urine of the patient with multiple myeloma free light chains (Bence-Jones protein) are present in addition to β_2 microglobulin reflecting tubular damage.

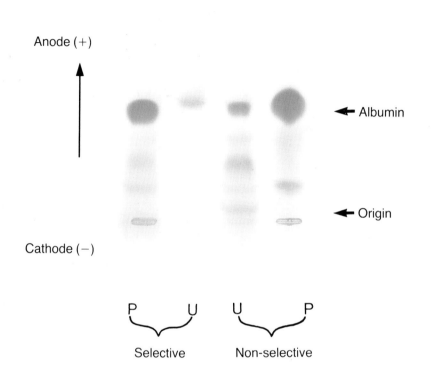

40 Electrophoresis of urine (U) and plasma (P) on cellulose acetate. The selectivity of proteinuria may be gauged by comparing the electrophoretic pattern of urine and blood. In non-selective proteinuria the slower-moving larger-molecular-weight proteins are seen in both the plasma and urine. In selective proteinuria only albumin is seen in significant amounts in the urine.

Table 19: Proteins in the urine

PROTEIN	MOLECULAR WEIGHT	NORMAL 24-HOUR URINE EXCRETION	CLEARANCE (% GFR)
Total	Variable	<250 mg	–
Albumin	65,000	<200 mg	0.02
β_2 Microglobulin	11,800	200 μg	80
K light chains	22,000	2.6 mg	8
λ light chains	22,000	1.5 mg	8
Lysozyme	14,500	1 mg	

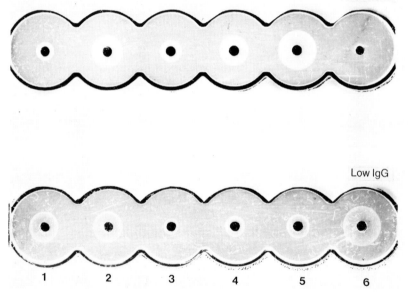

41 **Protein selectivity.** Serum and urine IgG and transferrin concentration are measured by radial diffusion from the central well into agarose containing specific antibody. The diameter of the precipitation ring is proportional to the concentration. Well 1 contains serum, well 2 contains urine, wells 3, 4 and 5 are standards. Well 6 is standard IgG, with a blank transferrin. In the above example, proteinuria is non-selective.

Selectivity index

In some clinical situations it is helpful to assess the selectivity of glomerular proteinuria. This is easily done by collecting a few millilitres of blood and urine. The concentration of IgG and transferrin is measured in both samples (**41**). Selectivity is the ratio of the clearance of IgG (molecular weight 150,000) to that of transferrin (molecular weight 88,000).

$$Selectivity\ Index = \frac{Clearance\ IgG}{Clearance\ of\ Transferrin}$$

$$= \frac{UIgG \times Ptr}{PIgG \times Utr}$$

where UIgG = Urine concentration of IgG
PIgG = Plasma concentration of IgG
Utr = Urine concentration of Transferrin
Ptr = Plasma concentration of Transferrin.

Selectivity can also be gauged from cellulose acetate electrophoresis of urine (**40**).

Highly selective proteinuria occurs when the selectivity index is less than 0.2. The principal clinical value of this index is in the assessment of the child with nephrotic syndrome. Highly selective proteinuria suggests the minimal change lesion producing the nephrotic syndrome. A trial of steroid therapy may then be given without the necessity of confirmation by a prior renal biopsy.

Microproteinuria

Methods: Proteinuria of less than 300mg/24 hours may indicate early renal disease. It can be detected by any of the following techniques:

1. Coomasie blue dye binding technique which relies on the protein error phenomenon as described with the stick tests (page 18).
2. Rocket immunoelectrophoresis, in which the urine containing albumin migrates into a gel impregnated with specific antibody to human albumin, under the influence of a steady electric current.
3. Specific radioimmunoassay for albumin.
4. Polyacrylamide gel electrophoresis of urine (qualitative).

Normal values:	Dye Binding method	< 50mg/24 hrs.
	Rocket technique	< 25mg/24 hrs.
	Radioimmunoassay	< 15mg/24 hrs.

Significance: Microproteinuria is below the limit of detection by stick tests and the biuret method. It is a useful screening test for early diabetic glomerular disease, and may also be of value in other states of hyperperfusion including hypertension. In the diabetic, microproteinuria has been shown to reflect poor early control, and can in fact be reduced by tight regulation of blood sugar. It may have some value in predicting those patients who will progress to overt clinical diabetic nephropathy.

Pigmenturia

Haemoglobinuria
Free haemoglobin is filtered at the glomerulus and appears in the urine. The peripheral blood film may show evidence of intravascular haemolysis (microangiopathic haemolytic anaemia). Plasma free haemoglobin will be elevated and the plasma haptoglobulin concentration reduced. Plasma lactate dehydrogenase will also be elevated, as this enzyme is released from damaged red cells. If haemoloysis is gross, as in a mismatched blood transfusion, plasma is pink on centrifugation of a few millilitres of peripheral blood. Haemoglobin is rapidly taken up by the tubular cells and converted to haemosiderin. If the urine deposit is stained using the Prussian blue reaction, then haemosiderinuria can be diagnosed. Urine spectroscopy can confirm the presence of haemoglobin in urine and differentiate it from myoglobin (Table 20).

Myoglobinuria
Myoglobin is of a smaller molecular weight than haemoglobin and is more rapidly filtered by the kidney. It is seldom possible to detect free myoglobin in the plasma. The presence of severe muscle damage capable of producing myoglobinuria is suggested by the finding of a grossly elevated creatine phosphokinase in the blood. Damaged muscles bind calcium and release potassium, purines and creatinine. In acute rhabdomyolysis there is a characteristic biochemical profile (Table 20) which can be compared to that associated with haemoglobinuria. Characteristically, urine containing myoglobin is red when fresh and turns black on standing. A simple side-room test can be used to distinguish haemoglobinuria from myoglobinuria (**42**). Again, urine spectroscopy will confirm the presence of myoglobinuria.

Table 20: Haemoglobinuria and myoglobinuria

	Haemoglobin	Myoglobin
Molecular wt.:	75,000	17,800
% Clearance of creatinine:	< 5	75

	Haemoglobinuria	Myoglobinuria
Cause:	Intravascular haemolysis	Rhabdomyolysis
Diagnosis:	↑ Plasma lactate dehydrogenase	↑ Plasma creatine phosphokinase
	Pink plasma: ↑ Plasma free haemoglobin	Normal plasma: Free plasma myoglobin not detectable (freely filtered at glomerulus)
	↓ Plasma haptoglobulin	Hypocalcaemia
	Abnormal peripheral blood film	Hyperkalaemia Hyperuricaemia
	↑ Unconjugated bilirubin (late)	Plasma creatinine > Urea
		Acidosis
Spectroscopy	Oxyhaemoglobin 540-α Oxyhaemoglobin 578-β Carboxyhaemoglobin 570-α	Oxymyoglobin 542-β Oxymyoglobin 582-α Carboxymyoglobin 578-α

(Wavelengths of absorption peaks in nm and absorption bands indicated by Greek letters.)

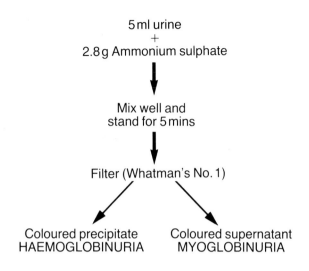

5 ml urine
+
2.8 g Ammonium sulphate

Mix well and
stand for 5 mins

Filter (Whatman's No. 1)

Coloured precipitate Coloured supernatant
HAEMOGLOBINURIA   MYOGLOBINURIA

42 Differentiation of myoglobinuria from haemoglobinuria

Urinary enzymes

Three enzymes are commonly measured in the urine:

1. NAG (N-Acetyl-β –D– glucosaminidase)
2. γGT (γ Glutamyl transferase)
3. Lysozyme.

All are widely distributed in various tissues but their urinary excretion can provide information about proximal tubular damage. Both NAG and γGT are present in significant quantities in the proximal tubule and will be released into the urine in disease states in which there is proximal tubular damage. Both are high molecular weight compounds and are not filtered normally by the glomerulus. Lysozyme is, however, a low molecular weight protein (MW 14,500) which is normally freely filtered by the glomerulus and virtually completely reabsorbed by the proximal tubule. Very high plasma levels may therefore be associated with increased urinary excretion although the tubular maximal reabsorptive capacity for lysozyme far exceeds usual plasma concentrations.

Plasma γGT is widely used as an index of liver disease. Plasma lysozyme serves as a marker for monocytic and myelomonocytic leukaemia. Plasma levels are not used to assess renal function although plasma lysozyme levels will rise as GFR falls.

The urinary excretion levels of these enzymes are helpful and provide a valuable and sensitive index of tubular damage (Table 21).

Urinary NAG

Assay: Fluorimetric assays using 4-methyl-umbelliferyl substrates are available and can be adapted for AutoAnalyzers.

Normal values: As for γGT, urinary NAG is usually corrected for creatinine excretion. A spot sample is usually sufficient, and the results are expressed as follows:

$$\frac{NAG\ activity}{Creatinine\ concentration} = \begin{array}{l} 53\text{–}884\ \mu IU/l/mg\ urine\ creatinine. \\ (6\text{–}134\ \mu IU/l/\mu mol\ urine\ creatinine) \end{array}$$

Table 21: Conditions associated with increased urinary excretion of NAG, lysozyme and β_2 microglobulin

Acute tubular damage	Ischaemia
	Toxins: Heavy Metals
	Drugs: Aminoglycosides
	X-ray contrast media
	Hypokalaemia
Upper tract infection (acute pyelonephritis)	
Congenital tubular disorders, e.g. Fanconi's Syndrome	
Acute renal allograft rejection	
Interstitial nephritis	

Urinary γGT

Assay: A synthetic chromogenic substrate (γ glutamyl-p-nitro-anilide) is used to measure γGT.

Normal values: To allow for alterations in GFR, urinary concentration of γGT should be expressed as a ratio of the creatinine clearance. This allows for the fact that the amount of γGT present in normal urine is proportional to the mass of functioning nephrons.

$$\frac{Total\ 24\text{-}hour\ \gamma\ GT\ (U/24\ hr)}{Creatinine\ clearance\ (ml/min)} = 0.17\text{–}0.52$$

Urinary Lysozyme
Lysozyme is an enzyme that breaks up bacterial cell walls. It is present in

the lysosomes of phagocytic cells and tubular epithelial cells.

Lysoplate assay: Lysozyme is allowed to diffuse from a well cut in agarose gel containing a suspension of cell wall constituents and the degree of lysis measured.

> *Normal values:* Plasma: *1.9–6.1µg/ml*
>   Urine: *1µg/ml*

An elevated urinary lysozyme gives the same information as an elevated urinary β_2 microglobulin but the assay for lysozyme is considerably cheaper.

β_2 Microglobulin (β_2M)

Structure
β_2 microglobulin is a ubiquitous polypeptide (100 amino-acids, MW 11,800) present on the surface of all nucleated cells. β_2M is an integral part of histo-compatibility locus antigen complex. Approximately 200mg of β_2M is produced every day.

Renal handling: β_2M is freely filtered at the glomerulus with a clearance of 80% of that of endogenous creatinine. There is avid proximal tubular reabsorption of β_2M, such less than 0.1% of the filtered load is excreted in the urine in normal subjects.

Plasma β_2M
Provided that production remains constant, the plasma β_2M concentration is a good guide to overall renal function, providing much the same information as the plasma creatinine concentration. Increased production and increased shedding of β_2M into the plasma may occur in various conditions such as the following:

1. Myelo-proliferative disorders.
2. Chronic inflammatory diseases.
3. Active liver disease.

Plasma β_2M may be used as a guide to overall renal function if the above conditions are excluded.

Urinary β_2M
Normals excrete less than 370µg of β_2M/24 hours. Increased urinary

β_2M is produced by lesions affecting the proximal tubule. It has proved difficult to demonstrate saturation of the tubular reabsorptive capacity for β_2M, so that an elevated urinary β_2M is likely to be due to proximal tubular damage rather than over-production and saturation of tubular reabsorptive pathways. Some amino-acids (lysine, ornithine and arginine) do compete with β_2M for tubular reabsorption, and urinary excess may lead to increased urinary excretion of β_2M.

Assay

β_2M is readily assayed by radio-immunoassay techniques using commercially available kits (Phadebas β_2 micro test, Pharmacia Ltd.).

> *Normal values:*   *Plasma:*   *0.8–2.4mg/l*
>   *Urine:*   *30–370 μg/24 hours*
>   *or 50μg/mmol creatinine*
> *Haemodialysis patients: plasma β_2M : 10–90mg/l.*

β_2M is rapidly degraded in acid urine. Prior to urine collection the patient should be given 4g sodium bicarbonate orally the night before, followed by 1g every six hours during the subsequent 24-hour urine collection period.

Applications

Urine β_2M is a semi-quantitative marker of tubular damage produced by various drugs, toxins and diseases:–

1. Screening for Balkan endemic nephropathy.
2. Monitoring renal transplants. With good immediate graft function plasma and urine β_2M fall to normal by five days. During an acute rejection episode there is a rise in plasma β_2M, followed a day or so later by a rise in urinary β_2M. Some workers suggest that the plasma β_2M rises before the plasma creatinine. Inter-current infection may produce a rise in plasma β_2M, so the test is not entirely specific. In primary non-function due to acute tubular necrosis, a fall in plasma β_2M heralds recovery as the recovering proximal tubular cells catabolise β_2M.
3. Differential diagnosis of upper from lower tract infection. In active bacterial pyelonephritis both plasma and urinary β_2M are elevated. Levels remain normal in cystitis.
4. Under the regulations governing Health and Safety at Work, workers exposed to heavy metals should be screened for increased urinary β_2M.

4: SPECIALISED INVESTIGATIONS: FURTHER RADIOLOGY

Renal arteriography

Method
Renal arteriography is performed by introducing a catheter into the femoral artery and injecting a large volume of contrast rapidly by a mechanical pump. This produces a free flush arteriogram. The catheter is then advanced to catheterise first one and then the other renal artery, and further injections of contrast are given to produce selective renal arteriograms.

Complications
The technique is unpleasant and invasive. In older patients there is a risk of dissection and of producing an embolus from a dislodged atheroma plaque. Local complications may occur at the site of the arterial puncture. Large volumes of X-ray contrast medium are potentially nephrotoxic. The use of the newer non-ionic contrast is preferred. Excellent pictures can be obtained with small volumes of contrast by using the newer digital subtraction techniques.

Indications
An arteriogram gives a precise anatomical demonstration of the vasculature of the kidney (Table 22, 43). The presence or absence of major vessel disease (44) and the presence of an abnormal tumour circulation (45) can be demonstrated. During an arteriogram there are therapeutic possibilities. Balloon dilatation of a renal artery stenosis may be undertaken (46–48). It is possible to embolise a bleeding point after a renal biopsy (49) or to embolise a vascular tumour prior to surgery via the catheter in the renal artery. Bleeding from a polycystic kidney can also be demonstrated and sometimes stopped by embolisation (50).

Renal vein venography

Method
A catheter is advanced via the femoral vein in the groin to the inferior vena cava. A free flush venogram is carried out to demonstrate any major

lesion (clot or compression) of the inferior vena cava (IVC). Each renal vein is then catheterised in turn. If necessary, a simultaneous selective renal artery catheterisation with adrenalin infusion can be carried out to reduce renal perfusion, in order to improve the quality of the venogram picture.

Complications
Local vessel damage may occur, but the venogram is relatively safe. A major pulmonary embolus can be precipitated in the presence of a fresh iliofemoral or IVC thrombosis.

Indications
The main value of the renal vein venogram is in collecting blood samples for renin assays in the investigation of hypertension. Great care must be taken in the labelling and handling of samples lest they be wasted. In addition to demonstrating the presence or absence of a renal vein thrombosis (54–56), the venogram may reveal the presence of tumour extension from a hypernephroma (Table 23). CT scanning provides the same information but less invasively.

Table 22: Indications for renal arteriography

Investigation of hypertension:	Recent onset, severe hypertension
	Renal artery stenosis
	Fibromuscular hyperplasia
	Younger patients
Demonstration of tumour circulation	
Major vessel occlusion:	Embolus – rheumatic heart disease
	Occlusion – dissecting aneurysm
Trauma	
Investigation of non-functioning kidney	
Planning surgery to a single kidney	
Unexplained haematuria	
Diagnosis of macroscopic Polyarteritis Nodosum	
Therapeutic:	Balloon dilatation
	Embolisation of a bleeding point
	Embolisation of vascular tumour
Investigation of a potential live kidney donor	
Investigation of a poorly functioning renal transplant	
	Chronic (vascular) rejection
	Renal artery stenosis

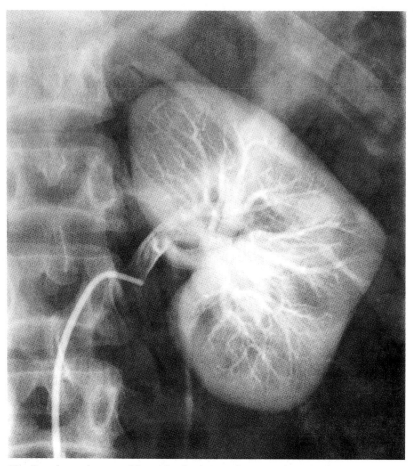

43 Renal arteriogram: Normal selective study. Note that the fine branches of the renal artery extend almost to the edge of the renal outline. The renal veins may also be demonstrated and a pyelogram appears on later films.

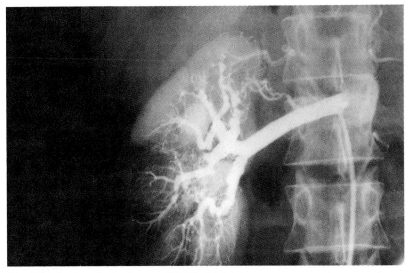

44 Selective renal arteriogram (PAN). Multiple aneurysms on the major intra-renal arteries are demonstrated in this patient with the macroscopic variety of polyarteritis nodosa (PAN).

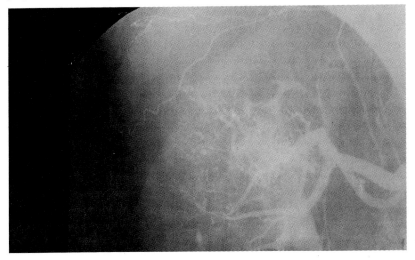

45 Selective renal arteriogram: Hypernephroma. Pathological vessels produced by the tumour circulation characteristic of a hypernephroma will distinguish it from a simple cyst (**52**).

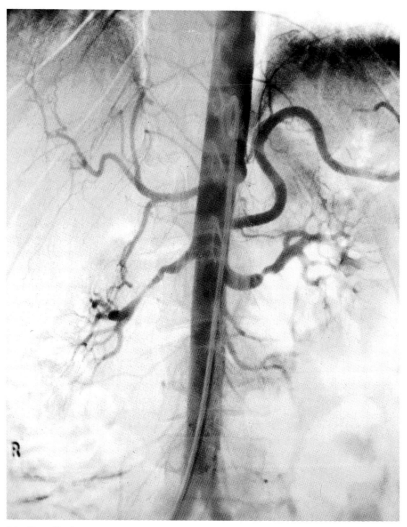

46 Free flush arteriogram (subtraction films): Fibromuscular dysplasia. There is bilateral renal artery stenosis due to fibromuscular hyperplasia, worse on the right. Balloon angioplasty was carried out (see **47** and **48**).

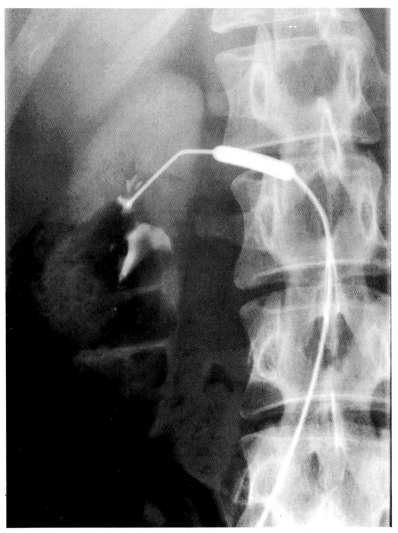

47 Balloon catheter. Dilatation of renal artery stenosis (**46** and **48**) can be carried out via a percutaneous approach using balloon catheters such as the one shown here.

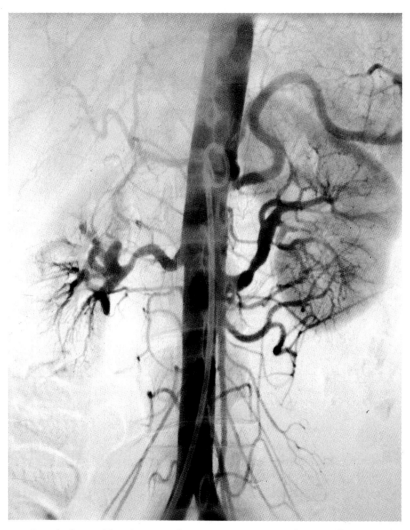

48 Post balloon dilatation: renal artery stenosis secondary to fibromuscular hyperplasia (subtraction films) compare with **46.**

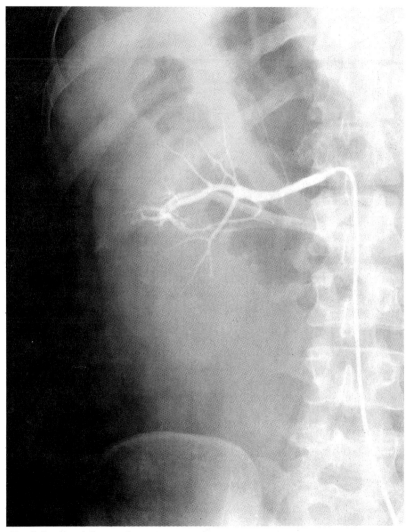

49 Selective right renal arteriogram: Arteriovenous fistula. The renal vein can be seen filling. This study was carried out after a renal biopsy which was complicated by a severe haemorrhage. The fistula was successfully embolised at this study and the bleeding stopped.

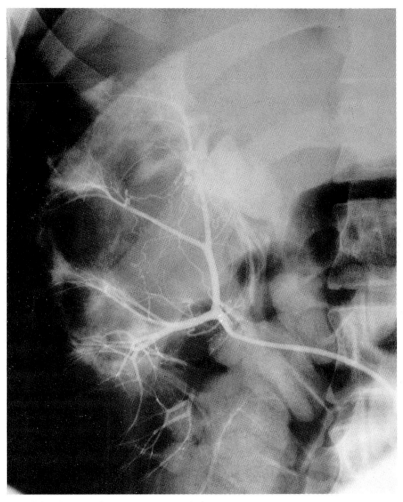

50 Selective renal arteriogram: Polycystic kidneys. Leak of contrast into the upper calyces is demonstrated, which accounted for heavy haematuria. Embolisation of the upper pole artery stopped the bleeding.

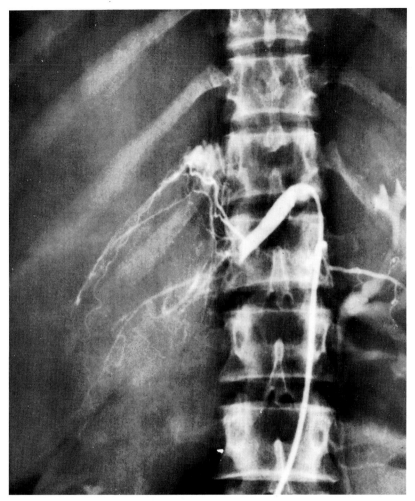

51 Renal arteriogram: Embolus. Late films from a selective right renal angiogram. This film demonstrates occlusion of the main right renal artery with a good illustration of the blood supply to the right suprarenal gland. On the left the contrast can be seen in the renal pelvis, calyces and ureter because of the lateness of the films. The left side is normal. The right kidney has infarcted after an acute embolus in a patient with severe rheumatic mitral valve disease.

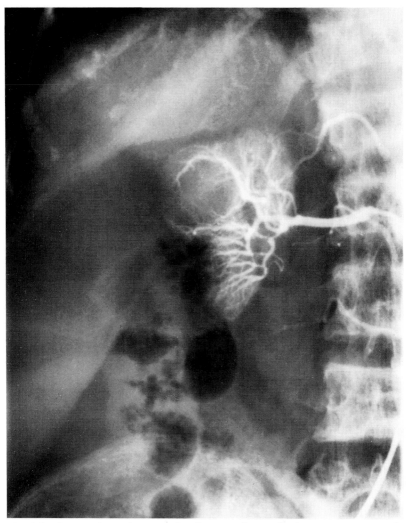

52 Selective renal arteriogram: Simple cyst. This study demonstrates a simple cyst in a small, contracted 'end stage' kidney. There is no pathological tumour circulation (compare with **45**).

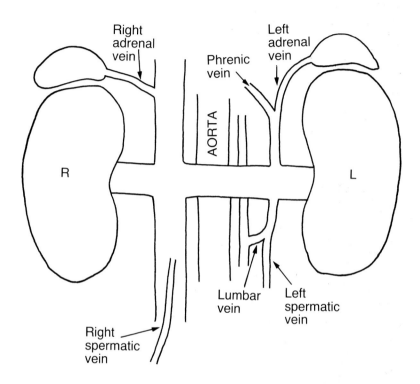

53 Renal venous drainage. It is important to remember that anomalies of renal venous drainage are quite common.

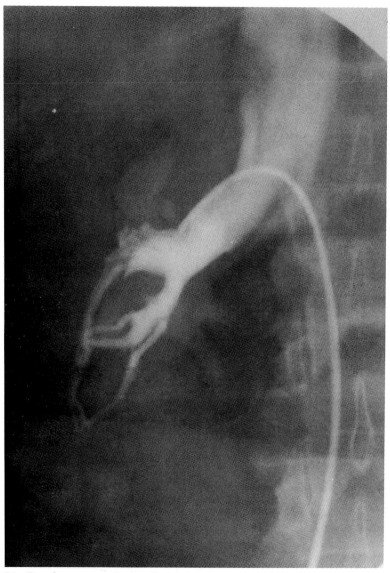

54 Renal venogram: Normal. Contrast has entered the small intrarenal branches of the renal vein. There are no filling defects and streaming of blood can be seen as the effluent from the right kidney joins the IVC.

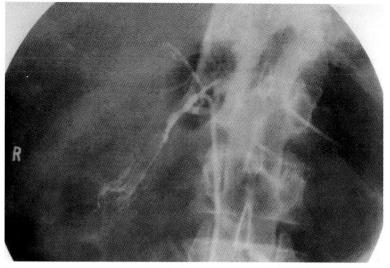

55 Renal venogram: Thrombosis. Extensive thrombosis in the main right renal vein has been demonstrated.

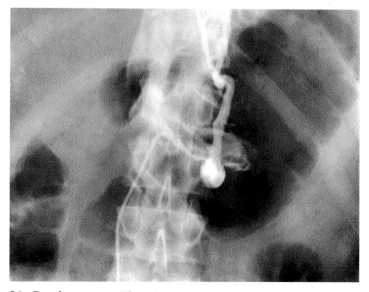

56 Renal venogram: Thrombosis with collaterals. Extensive thrombosis fills the left renal vein and contrast has entered collateral channels (see **53**).

Table 23: Indications for renal vein venography

1 Selective renal vein sampling for renin
2 Detection of renal vein thrombosis:
  Nephrotic syndrome
  Hypovolaemic infants
3 Extension of tumour (Hypernephroma)
4 Renal transplant:
  Ipsilateral deep vein thrombosis, with extension to the
  transplant vein

Isotope scans of the kidney

Scanning techniques have improved greatly over the last ten years. Improvements have meant that images are now of such good quality that in some instances it may be preferable to scan before carrying out an IVU. The techniques of scanning and conventional radiology should not be viewed as competing but as being able to shed light on each other's grey areas. Discussion with the radiologists and nuclear medicine departments will save valuable time and help to establish the best sequence of investigations in a given patient. A good example of this decision-making process is in the assessment of a patient with acute renal failure. Most agree that an urgent ultrasound and KUB are mandatory, but what to do next? It may be appropriate to do no further renal imaging or to do an emergency IVU or DTPA renogram. The decision depends on what is the likely cause of the renal failure – nephrotoxins, obstruction, ischaemia, infarction, etc.

The principal areas in which isotope scanning can be of value are listed in Table 24. One great advantage of isotopes is that they still give clear pictures in the obese subject or through gas-filled loops of overlying bowel. Scanning is a non-invasive way of demonstrating renal perfusion, gross disease of major blood vessels, and the vascularity of areas of the kidney or suspected mass lesions. Suspicious lesions will need the greater detail that a selective renal arteriogram can provide.

An IVU will not give information about renal function. Assessing relative function from an IVU is often very misleading. An isotope renogram (DMSA) gives a much better indication of the distribution of functioning renal tissue (58).

Static imaging

Method: 2mCi of Technetium labelled DMSA (dimercaptosuccinic acid) is given intravenously. The DMSA binds to tubular cells (probably to SH groups in the proximal tubule). Uptake by the kidney indicates the presence of viable renal tissue. Gamma camera pictures are usually taken three to four hours after the intravenous injection, by which time approximately 70% of the administered dose is bound to the kidney. It is also possible to display the activity of the kidney for the first 60 seconds after a good intravenous bolus by recording serial one-second frames. This provides an image of the vascular phase.

Interpretation of results: The ^{99m}Tc DMSA scan provides a simple and reliable non-invasive method of assessing the individual contribution of each kidney to total renal function (57). It is a valuable test and may prevent the surgeon from carrying out a nephrectomy when considerable renal function remains on the diseased side (>20%). It can tell a surgeon which of the two kidneys to operate on first. A demonstration of 'cold', poorly perfused areas of non-functioning renal tissue in a kidney full of calculi can guide the surgeon's operative approach. In children or young adults with reflux and suspected chronic pyelonephritis (reflux nephropathy), cortical scars can be clearly demonstrated. Similarly, cortical infarcts from emboli are easily visualised (58). DMSA scans may fail to distinguish cysts from tumours as both can have areas of non-functioning renal tissue.

Indications: ^{99m}Tc DMSA scans are particularly helpful prior to surgery to guide surgical approach and to ensure that potentially useful functioning renal tissue is not unnecessarily removed (Table 24).

Dynamic Imaging

Method: Technetium labelled DTPA (diethylenetriamine penta-acetic acid) or ^{131}I labelled hippuran may be used. DTPA is in many ways preferable as it is more easily obtained. DTPA is handled by glomerular filtration whilst hippuran is filtered and secreted. Hippuran is cleared very rapidly. This means that it is difficult to get a clear impression of a vascular phase without giving very large doses. Whichever compound is used, the elimination of the agent is followed by gamma camera pictures and computer plotting of activity over the kidneys, bladder and vascular pool (59). The radiation dose with either agent is smaller than that associated with the conventional IVU. The information obtained from these scans is similar to that obtained from the IVU but without its more precise anatomical definition. By counting over the bladder before and after micturition and counting the activity of voided urine, an accurate measure of residual urine in the bladder can be made. It is also possible to demonstrate vesico-ureteric reflux, but a micturating cysto-urethrogram is the preferred investigation for suspected reflux.

Interpretation of results: The normal renogram has three phases. The first phase is the vascular phase, the second corresponds to an accumulation of the isotope within the nephron and is termed the 'secretory phase'. The third phase documents the excretion of the agent from the kidney (**59**). It is crucial that the injection of DTPA be given as a good, sharp bolus, otherwise the first phase spreads and obscures this pattern. Obstruction produces a delay in the third phase (**60**) and in the acute situation there may be a slight increase in renal blood flow. Renal artery stenosis (**62**) produces a prolonged uptake of tracer, with delay in reaching the peak of the second phase. Excretion is prolonged. Chronic parenchymal disease produces flattening of the second phase. In acute tubular necrosis there is a reduction in blood flow and a flattening of phase II and phase III (**60**).

Indications: The DTPA renogram is a valuable screening investigation and may be used for follow-up studies to assess response to surgical treatment for obstruction (Table 24). In many respects the investigation is complementary to the IVU. In patients with dilated collecting systems, excretion may be slow because of pooling rather than true obstruction. This situation may be resolved by giving an intravenous bolus of frusemide (0.5–1mg/kg/body weight) at 20 minutes. If a marked wash-out effect is seen (**61, 63**) then obstruction is unlikely to be present. If the half-time ($T\frac{1}{2}$) of the wash-out after frusemide is seven minutes or less, then obstruction is most unlikely. A $T\frac{1}{2}$ of 12 minutes or more suggests the presence of obstruction.

Table 24: Indications for isotope renography

^{99m}Tc DMSA	^{99m}Tc DTPA
(Dimercaptosuccinic acid)	(Diethylenetriamine-penta-acetic acid)

Static imaging

Cortical scars:
    Chronic pyelonephritis
    Infarcts
    Calculus disease

Divided renal function tests

Non-functioning kidney

Ectopic kidney

Vascularity of mass lesions

Diagnosis of pseudo-tumour of
   Columns of Bertin

Obese subjects

Neo-natal kidney imaging

Screening for segmental renal
   artery stenosis

Dynamic imaging

Major vessel disease

Obstruction or dilatation

Acute renal failure: perfusion

Screening hypertensive patients

Renal transplant monitoring

Obese subjects

Follow up, e.g.:
    Post angioplasty
    Repair of PUJ obstruction
    During treatment for TB

Residual bladder volume

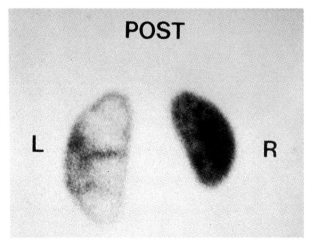

57 ^{99m}Tc DMSA Scan (posterior view) demonstrating residual function in the hydronephrotic remnant of a chronically obstructed left kidney. L = 10%, R = 90% of total renal function.

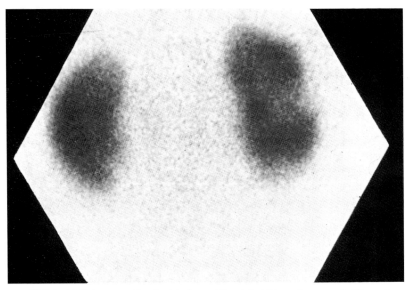

58 ^{99m}Tc DMSA scan: **Cortical infarct.** The left kidney is normal. There is a deep wedge-shaped defect in the cortex of the right kidney caused by an embolus, producing an infarct.

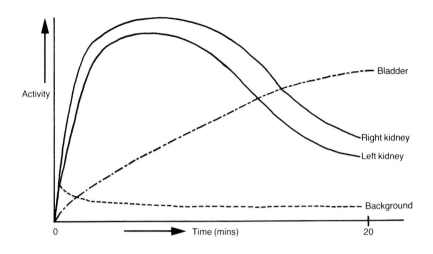

59 ^{99m}Tc DTPA renogram: Elimination curves – normal.

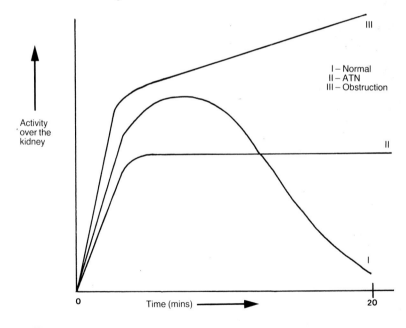

60 ^{99m}Tc DTPA renogram: Elimination curves – abnormal.

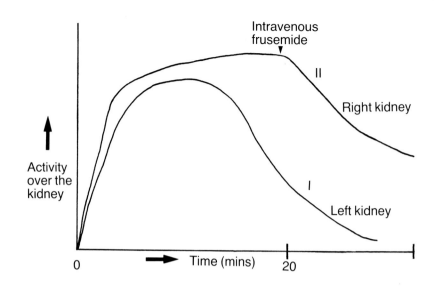

61 ^{99m}Tc DTPA Renogram – elimination curves – dilatation. Trace I from the left kidney is normal. Trace II shows delayed excretion from the right kidney which washes out promptly after intravenous frusemide. This finding implies a dilated but non-obstructed renal pelvis and calyces on the right and indicates that an operation would be inappropriate.

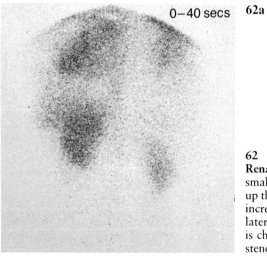

0–40 secs **62a**

62 ^{99m}Tc DTPA renogram: Renal artery stenosis. Note the small right kidney which takes up the DTPA slowly and shows increased concentration on the later pictures (B and C), which is characteristic of renal artery stenosis.

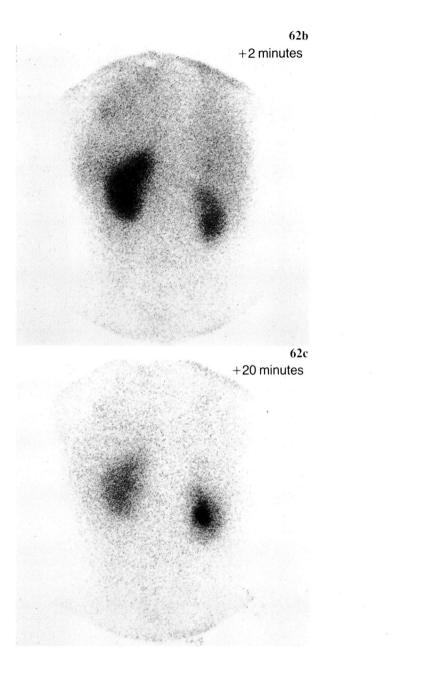

62b

+2 minutes

62c

+20 minutes

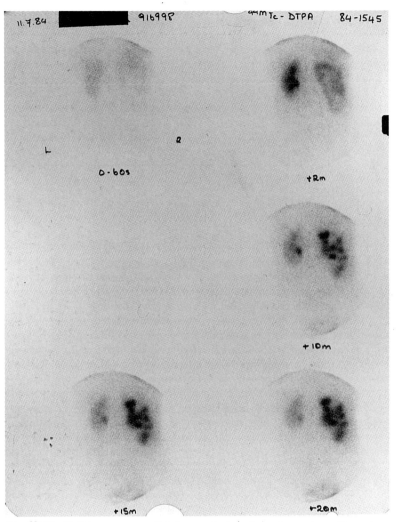

L   &   0-60s   +2m   +10m   +15m   +20m

63 ^{99m}Tc DTPA renogram: Pelvi-ureteric junction obstruction. Note the enlarged right kidney. Early images show a patchy nephrogram. Later images show this to be due to gross dilatation of the calyces and renal pelvis. At the end of the study isotope remains in the collecting system and pelvis, having been cleared from the left side. Despite I.V. frusemide no drainage from the right side occurs, signifying obstruction.

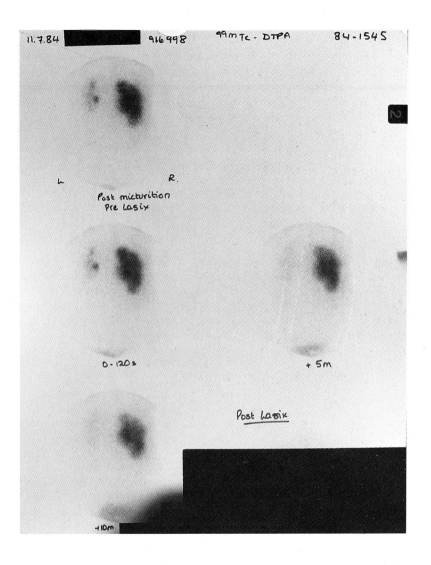

11.7.84 916 998 99m Tc - DTPA 84-1545

L R.

Post micturition
Pre Lasix

0 - 120 s + 5m

Post Lasix

+ 10m

Combined bone and renal imaging

The agent used for bone imaging is ^{99m}Tc labelled MDP (methylene diphosphonate). Some of the injected dose is cleared by the kidney, and a good renogram can be obtained, as with DTPA. Gamma camera pictures taken later demonstrate skeletal uptake. This provides an opportunity to do two studies for the price of one, and can be helpful in several situations, for example:

1. Renal tumours with bone secondaries
2. Carcinoma of the prostate with obstruction and bony deposits
3. Multiple myeloma
4. Renal transplants with suspected avascular necrosis of bone.

^{67}Gallium Scanning

^{67}Gallium is taken up by inflammatory tissues. Two to three days after the intravenous injection of 4.05mCi ^{67}Ga, gamma camera pictures are obtained of areas of potential interest. Preliminary studies indicate that active parenchymal infection of the kidneys (e.g. polycystic kidneys), perirenal infection and acute tubulo-interstitial nephritis can be detected by gallium scanning.

Micturating cysto-urethrogram

The purpose of this investigation is to demonstrate the presence or absence of reflux from the bladder up the ureters (**64**). The procedure will also demonstrate the adequacy of bladder emptying if the patient is able to co-operate. Good pictures of the urethra to demonstrate the presence of strictures or congenital valves may also be obtained (**65**).

Method: Under full aseptic conditions the bladder is catheterised and water-soluble radiographic contrast material is introduced to fill the bladder completely. Films are taken during filling. The catheter is then withdrawn and the patient asked to micturate. Further films are taken during voiding. Oblique films are necessary. Immediate post-micturition films assess the adequacy of bladder emptying and may also demonstrate reflux. It may be prudent to cover the procedure with a short course of antibiotics in patients particularly at risk of infection. Better views of the urethra can be obtained by an ascending urethrogram. If catheterisation of the bladder is not possible, contrast can be introduced by a suprapubic bladder puncture.

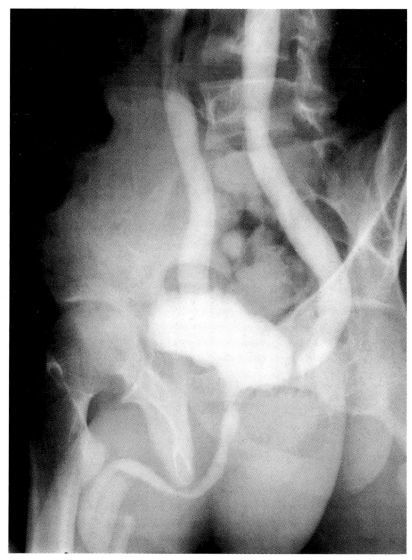

64 Micturating cysto-urethrogram (MCU): Reflux. Oblique view of an MCU demonstrating gross bilateral vesico-ureteric reflux. The urethra is normal but the ureters are dilated and fill with contrast during micturition.

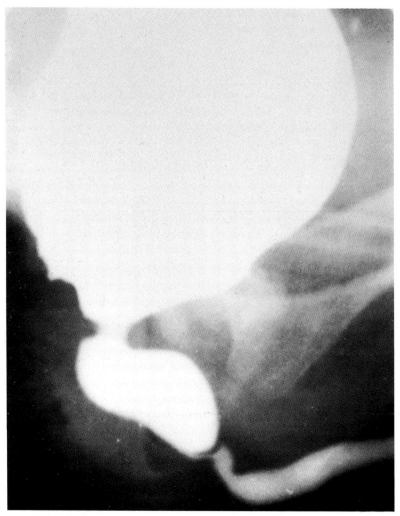

65 Micturating cysto-urethrogram: Urethral valves. This is a study carried out in a child which demonstrates obstruction due to urethral valves and dilatation of the proximal urethra and bladder. The IVU relating to this patient is shown in **66.**

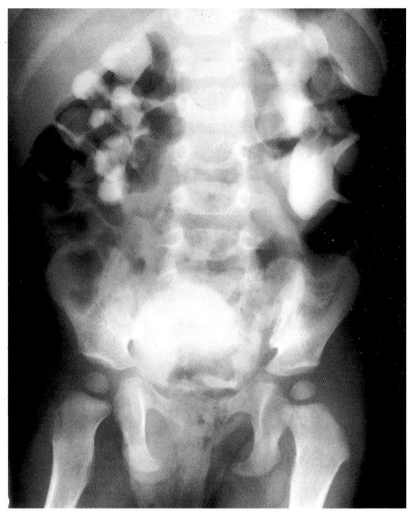

66 **IVU:** Bilateral hydronephrosis secondary to urethral valves. Gross bilateral hydronephrosis and bladder dilatation have been caused by obstruction from urethral valves (see **65**).

Antegrade pyelogram

Under X-ray screening or ultrasound control, a fine needle is introduced directly into a dilated calyx of the renal pelvis. Urine may then be aspirated for culture, cytology or biochemistry. Contrast is then instilled to demonstrate anatomy clearly. If obstruction is demonstrated (67), larger and larger catheters can be gradually introduced and then left in situ to drain the kidney. Subsequent definitive surgery may then be planned.

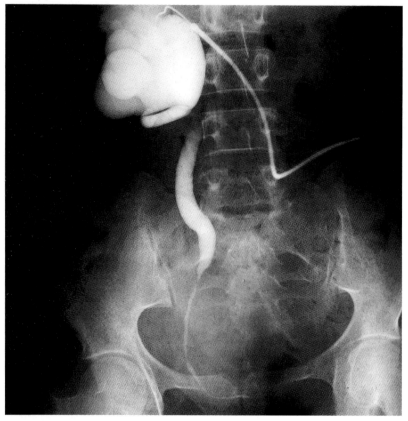

67 **Antegrade pyelogram:** Upper tract dilatation above a long stricture of the ureter has developed in a patient with carcinoma of the cervix with local spread producing external compression of the right ureter.

Retrograde pyelogram

A cystoscopy is performed under general anaesthetic and a ureteric catheter is placed in the lower end of the ureter under direct vision. A few millilitres of X-ray contrast material is then injected to outline the ureter (68). If necessary, samples of urine may be collected for culture or cytology. This technique enables precise localisation of obstruction (ureteric clot, calculi, tumour or stricture), and may delineate urothelial tumours not clearly demonstrated on an IVU. The risk of introducing infection, rupturing the ureter or producing trauma, with subsequent stricture formation, is very real. It is now no longer clinical practice to use this technique for divided renal function tests as isotope scanning techniques provide the necessary information non-invasively. Semi-permanent double pig-tail ureteric stents may be inserted to bypass ureteric strictures in suitable cases.

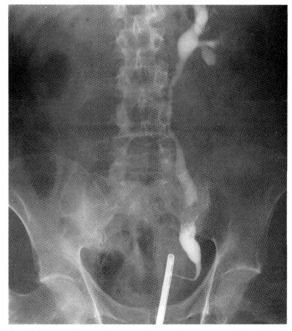

68 **Retrograde pyelogram: Ureteric tumour.** The large filling defect in the left ureter is due to a transitional cell carcinoma of the ureter.

CT Scanning of the renal tract

Computerised tomographic scanning is particularly valuable in demonstrating the retroperitoneal, perirenal and periureteric lesions that may be producing obstruction (**69–74**). CT is also valuable for the investigation of masses or suspected tumours and should be undertaken early. Staging of tumours is more accurately done by CT than by ultrasound. It is usual to give a dose of intravenous contrast to highlight the kidneys during the investigation. Whether or not a lesion enhances with contrast may aid the differential diagnosis.

The pelvis is difficult to visualise clearly with ultrasound or IVU, but CT scanning will clearly demonstrate the anatomy and is therefore of value in the assessment of prostatic, bladder and cervical tumours (**70, 74**). CT scanning is also helpful at showing direct extension of the tumour. Less expensive techniques (IVU, ultrasound, cyst puncture) are probably as reliable and are therefore still necessary when it comes to resolving the probable nature of an intrarenal space-occupying lesion. Obstruction is still best diagnosed by ultrasound or an IVU.

Images can be reformatted in sagittal and coronal displays. This can be helpful to demonstrate a phaeochromocytoma or adrenal tumour.

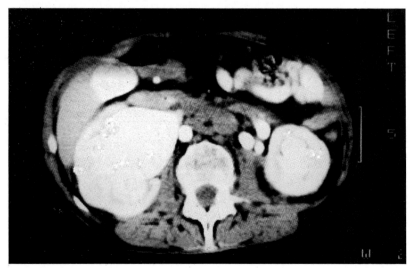

69   CT scan: Bilateral obstruction. This scan was taken after IV contrast. Gross bilateral obstruction and hydronephrosis have been demonstrated. Subsequent 'cuts' through the pelvis demonstrated the cause of the obstruction (see **70**).

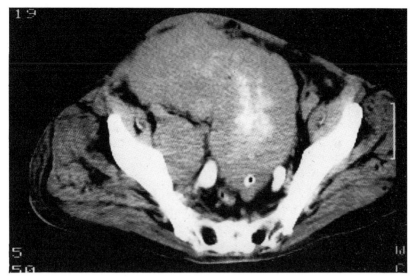

70 CT scan: Bladder tumour. The scan of the pelvis shows a massive bladder tumour extending anteriorly from the bladder. A small amount of contrast is seen in the much reduced lumen of the bladder. A large mass of malignant nodes is present on the right of the pelvis.

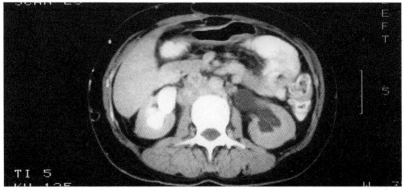

71 CT scan: Acute obstruction. This scan was carried out after intravenous contrast to enhance the kidneys and also during an ascending venogram. Marked bilateral obstruction is present with a negative pyelogram on the left side. The small dots of contrast at the front and right side of the film represent contrast in dilated venous collaterals. Thrombosis can be seen in the inferior vena cava. Lower cuts (**72**) confirm the presence of a retroperitoneal mass involving the ureters and inferior vena cava.

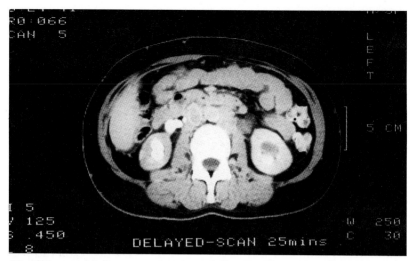

72 CT scan: Malignant retroperitoneal fibrosis. Clot within the inferior vena cava and contrast in anterior abdominal wall collateral vessels can be seen. There is a mass of retroperitoneal tissue surrounding the inferior vena cava and obstructing both ureters.

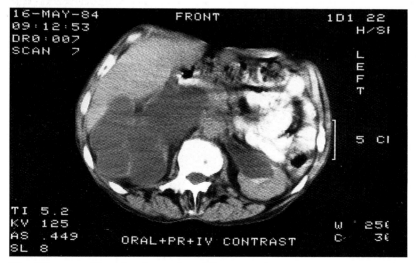

73 CT scan: Chronic obstruction. The scan shows gross hydronephrotic changes in both kidneys with a marked degree of loss of cortical tissue on the right. Lower cuts (**74**) demonstrated the cause of the obstruction.

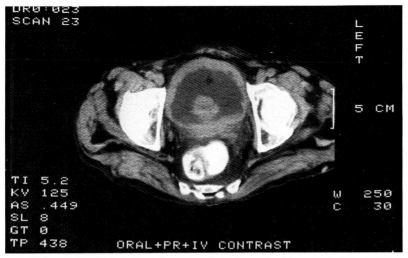

74   CT scan: Benign prostatic hypertrophy. The scan of the pelvis shows a thick walled dilated bladder. The central shadow within the bladder represents gross prostatic hypertrophy. There was no evidence of malignancy.

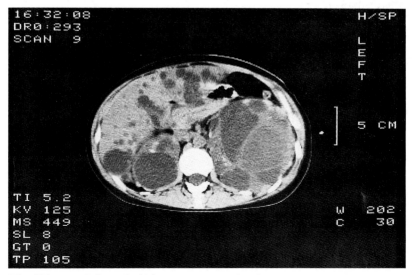

75   CT scan: Polycystic kidneys. Congenital polycystic kidneys and multiple cysts (asymptomatic) in the liver. The pancreas is seen clearly but is not involved in this particular patient.

Digital subtraction angiography (DSA) of the kidney

It is possible to obtain near arteriogram-quality pictures following an intravenous bolus of a small dose of contrast (30–50ml), with computerised subtraction analysis of X-ray images (76–78). This technique may be readily combined with renal vein venous sampling for renin in the investigation of hypertension and is also valuable in the renal transplant patient with poor graft function (Chapter 9). DSA is also of value in diabetics in whom large volumes of contrast should be avoided. It seems likely that the DSA will find a place in the screening of patients with severe hypertension looking for evidence of renal artery stenosis. Very high quality arteriograms can be produced using the DSA technique, with extremely small volumes of X-ray contrast after direct intra-arterial injections.

Lesions close to the aorta may not be clearly visualised. The rapid development of the nephrogram also restricts small vessel identification. Cardiac output must be good otherwise a sharp bolus of contrast does not reach the kidney.

76a

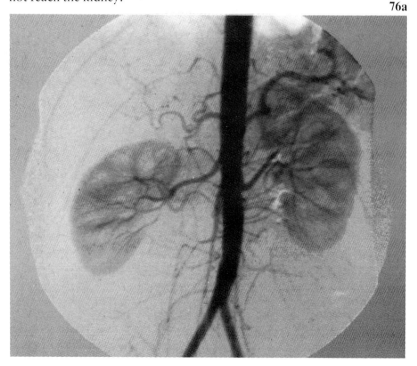

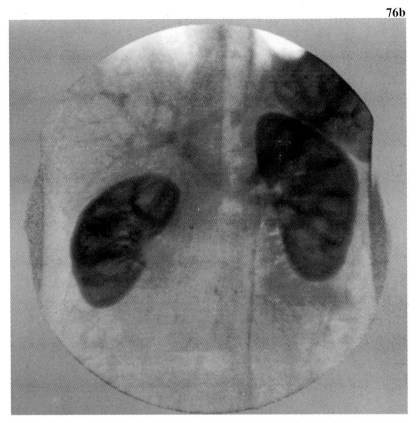

76   DSA Normal

a. Early pictures demonstrate normal renal arteries.
b. Later images produce an even nephrogram and may also demonstrate the renal veins.

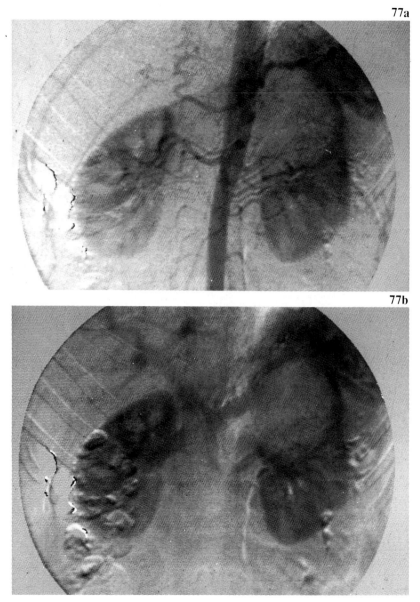

77 DSA: Simple cyst. The defect in the nephrogram is shown to be due to a simple cyst which lacks the abnormal vessels that would suggest a tumour. (a) early film, (b) late film.

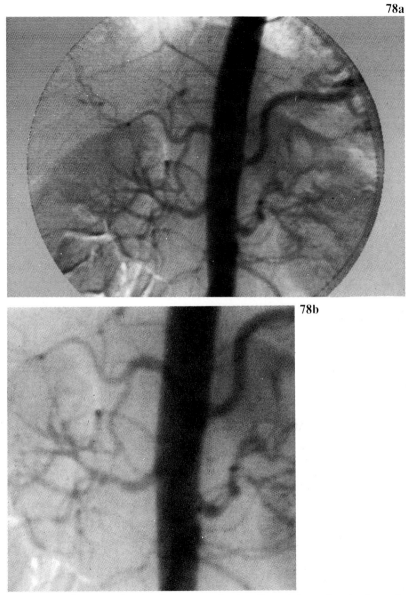

78 **DSA: Fibromuscular dysplasia.** Irregular beading of the major renal vessels is demonstrated, particularly on the magnified view (**b**).

5: SPECIALISED INVESTIGATIONS: RENAL TUBULE FUNCTION TESTS

Urinary Dilution

Physiology

The capacity to produce a dilute urine depends on the reabsorption of solutes without water in the ascending limb of the loop of Henlé. Patients with severe and progressive liver disease, cardiac failure and the nephrotic syndrome cannot produce a dilute urine. In these three conditions there is not only an increase in antidiuretic hormone but also avid reabsorption of sodium, chloride and water proximally, with reduced delivery of solute to the loop of Henlé. Such patients are prone to develop a dilutional hyponatraemia if allowed continued free access to water. In addition, as renal failure progresses patients with chronic renal disease show a fall in the ability of their kidneys to produce a dilute urine, along with the retention of nitrogenous waste products.

Method

Urinary dilution: The diluting capacity of the kidney may be estimated by a simple water loading test: the patient is asked to void. 1,000 to 1,500ml of water (20ml/kg body weight) is administered over 30 minutes. Half-hourly urine volumes are collected for the next five hours.

Normal values: More than 75% of the administered water load should be excreted within three hours. Urine osmolality should fall below 100mOsm/kg (Sp.Gr.<1.003).

A variety of factors may interfere with the dilution test such as nausea, vomiting, variations in gastric emptying and absorption, smoking and emotional factors.

Free water clearance: The ability of the kidney to make a dilute urine can be measured by assessing the free water clearance (CH_2O). 'Free water' is defined as the amount of water that must be added to or taken away from the urine to make it isotonic with plasma. A positive free water clearance means that the urine is more dilute than plasma, and a negative free water clearance means that the urine is more concentrated.

Osmolar clearance (Cosm) measures the volume of plasma that is cleared of osmotically active solutes in a unit time (minute). Looked at another way, Cosm is the volume of urine required to excrete all the solutes in the urine at an osmolality the same as that of plasma. Thus:

$$Cosm = \frac{Urine\ Osm \times urine\ volume\ (ml/min)}{Plasma\ Osm}$$

$$Free\ water\ clearance = Urine\ volume\ (ml/min) - Cosm\ (ml/min)$$

Interpretation of results
Formal testing of the capacity of the kidney to produce a dilute urine or the measurement of free water clearance is infrequently carried out in clinical practice. Conceptually it is very important, as the defect develops early in progressive liver disease, reflecting the deranged intrarenal haemodynamics that may culminate in the hepato-renal syndrome. It also helps to explain the marked dilutional hyponatraemia that is commonly found in cardiac failure.

Urine concentration

Formal testing of the ability to concentrate urine is not infrequently required in clinical medicine in the investigations of patients with polyuria. The main differential diagnosis in this clinical situation is between the patients with diabetes insipidus and those with compulsive water drinking. To distinguish between these two conditions sequential water deprivation followed by the administration of exogenous vasopressin should be carried out (Table 25).

Physiology
The kidney is able to produce a concentrated urine because of the interstitial medullary concentration gradient, selective and variable permeability of the collecting ducts to water and the release of ADH. The ascending limb of the loop of Henlé reabsorbs sodium and chloride without water and is responsible for the accumulation of solutes in the medullary interstitium. The unique hairpin arrangement of tubules and blood vessels ensures that the solutes remain trapped in the medulla. They may be 'washed out' in polyuric states when there is an increase in medullary blood flow as well as urine flow. The ascending limb of the loop of Henlé remains impermeable to water irrespective of the concentration of ADH. The collecting ducts, however, become permeable to water under the influence of ADH, which allows the reabsorption of water from their lumen as the ducts pass through the medulla, so producing a concentrated urine.

Method

6 p.m.: On the evening before the test, a baseline weight is recorded. Blood is taken for plasma urea, creatinine, electrolytes and osmolality. Urine osmolality is checked. No oral fluids are given after 12 midnight and until the conclusion of the test.

6 a.m.: On the following morning, the weighing is repeated. Fluid deprivation should be abandoned if the weight has dropped by more than 5% as dangerous dehydration will occur. The early morning urine samples are tested for osmolality. Further testing is unnecessary if the urine osmolality is already greater than 800mOsm/kg. Plasma urea, creatinine, electrolytes and osmolality are also checked.

7 a.m.: An intranasal insufflation of desmopressin (dDAVP) is given (20µg children, 40µg adults) into each nostril. Urine osmolality is tested hourly for the next six hours.

12 noon: Body weight is again checked. It is important to ensure that body weight does not fall by more than 5%.

Table 25: Investigation of polyuria

PATIENT	OVERNIGHT FLUID DEPRIVATION (URINE OSMOLALITY MOSM/KG)	RESPONSE TO EXOGENOUS VASOPRESSIN
Normal	> 900	No further increase
Complete Central Diabetes Insipidus	< 200	Marked increase in urine osmolality
Partial Central Diabetes Insipidus	< 500	Marked ($\geq 30\%$) increase in urine osmolality
Nephrogenic Diabetes Insipidus	< 300	No change
Compulsive water drinking	600–800	Minimal ($\leq 10\%$) rise in osmolality

Interpretation of results

A normal subject has a maximal output of ADH after water deprivation. Further exogenous vasopressin is ineffective. The patient with complete central diabetes insipidus lacks ADH and cannot respond to water deprivation, but makes a marked response to exogenous ADH. Because of the washout effect of polyuria on the interstitial medullary concentration gradient, maximum osmolality of the urine cannot be produced even with exogenous vasopressin. The patient with partial central diabetes insipidus still produces some ADH and can make a partial response to water deprivation, which is increased after the administration of exogenous ADH. In patients with nephrogenic diabetes insipidus, the distal tubule is unresponsive to ADH and they cannot respond to water deprivation. Similarly, they make no response to exogenous vasopressin.

Compulsive water drinkers produce polyuria which washes out the medullary concentration gradient. After a water deprivation test, they release maximal amounts of ADH. Nevertheless, they only produce suboptimal urine concentration. No further increase can occur after exogenous vasopressin.

Quality of the urine

General principles
In oliguric patients (<500ml/24 hrs) with acute renal failure, it is helpful to analyse the biochemical quality of the urine with respect to that of the plasma biochemistry.

In 'pre-renal' acute renal failure, the problem is inadequate perfusion of otherwise normal kidneys. In the patient who is hypovolaemic the kidney responds in a manner that is intended to improve its perfusion. In this situation, the kidney avidly conserves sodium and water, but continues to excrete urea and creatinine, making urine of high osmolality.

In intrinsic or established acute renal failure there is parenchymal disease of the kidney, the quality of the urine is poor and becomes more and more like that of unaltered glomerular filtrate.

These biochemical differences help to distinguish pre-renal acute renal failure (and the hepato-renal syndrome) from established acute tubular necrosis (Table 26). These guidelines only apply if the patient is oliguric and has not received diuretics. The important implication of these results is that if renal perfusion can be restored the patient with pre-renal renal failure may well recover normal function. As indicated in Table 26, the addition of urine microscopy further helps to define the underlying clinical situation.

Table 26: Quality of urine in oliguric acute renal failure

	PRE-RENAL	RENAL
Urinary Na (mmol/l)	< 10–20	> 20
Urinary urea (mmol/l)	> 250	< 150
Urine osmolality (mOsm/kg)	> 500	< 350
Urine / Plasma urea	> 20	< 10
Urine / Plasma creatinine	> 30	< 25
Urine / Plasma osmolality	> 1.5	< 1.1
Urine microscopy	Normal	Tubular epithelial cells ++ Tubular epithelial casts ++ Granular casts ++

Table 27: Sodium-losing nephropathies

Papillary necrosis:
    Analgesic nephropathy
    Sickle cell disease
    Diabetes Mellitus
Post obstruction
Polycystic disease (some cases)
Chronic pyelonephritis (some cases)
Recovery phase of acute tubular necrosis
Recovery after patchy cortical necrosis

Fractional Excretion of Sodium (FE_{Na})

The criteria for pre-renal ARF listed in Table 26 may not always be reliable. The derived index, the fractional excretion of sodium, is a better guide to the patient with pre-renal acute renal failure.

The fractional excretion of sodium =

$$\frac{Excreted\ Sodium}{Filtered\ Sodium}$$

$$Filtered\ Na = GFR \times PNa$$

$$= \frac{Ucr \times V}{Pcr} \times P\ Na.$$

$$Excreted\ Na = V \times U\ Na$$

$$FE_{Na}\% = \frac{U\ Na \times Pcr}{P\ Na \times Ucr} \times 100$$

Where V = *Urine volume*
$U\ Na$ = *Urine sodium concentration*
Ucr = *Urine creatinine concentration*
$P\ Na$ = *Plasma sodium concentration*
Pcr = *Plasma creatinine concentration*
Normal = *1–2%*
Pre-renal RF <1.0%
Intrinsic/Established RF >1.0%

The physiological principle behind the fractional excretion of sodium is the same as that underlying the spot urinary sodium concentration, i.e. an underperfused normal kidney avidly conserves sodium. FE_{NA} can be very low in the nephrotic syndrome, cirrhosis and heart failure. In ATN and in CRF, FE_{NA} may be high.

Inappropriate sodium losses

A variety of conditions are associated with sodium-losing states (Table 27). Recognition of salt-losers is important as sodium supplements help to preserve renal perfusion and GFR. If a patient is stabilised on 100mmol sodium diet for a few days urinary sodium losses should be no greater than 75–85mmol/day.

Inappropriate potassium losses

Abnormal loss of potassium in the urine is suggested by the finding of more than 20mmol potassium/24 hours in the urine when the plasma potassium is less than 3mmol/l.

Urine acidification tests

Excretion of acid

The process of metabolism produces an excess of hydrogen ions (H^+) that are ultimately excreted in the urine. Hydrogen ions appear in the urine as:

a Free H^+.
b Combined with buffer anions e.g. HPO_4^{--}, $H_2PO_4^{-}$.
c Combined with ammonia as ammonium (NH_4^+).

The term 'titratable acidity of the urine' refers to the sum of:

$$Free\ H^+ + Buffer\ anions\ H^+$$

It is measured by back titration with 0.1N sodium hydroxide.
Total net urine acid excretion is the sum of:

$$Titrable\ acidity + urine\ ammonium - urinary\ bicarbonate.$$

Types of renal tubular acidosis (RTA)

The patient has renal tubular acidosis if the urine pH is above 5.3 in the face of a systemic acidosis (plasma bicarbonate less than 22mmol/l). There are four main types of renal tubular acidosis:

Distal (Classical, Type I): The defect lies in the inability of the distal tubule to maintain a hydrogen ion gradient across the tubular lumen.

Proximal (Type II): The defect is impaired proximal tubular re-absorption of the filtered bicarbonate.

Mixed proximal and distal (Type III).

Hyporeninaemic (Type IV): Lack of renin leads to hypo-aldosteronism with reduced distal reabsorption of sodium, resulting in reduced hydrogen ion and potassium secretion.

The different types of renal tubular acidosis vary in their severity and associated clinical abnormalities. (Incomplete forms exist with urine pH in the alkaline range but without a systemic acidosis.) The mildest is Type IV, as urine may be acidic yet net excretion of acid is reduced. Patients with Type IV RTA usually have a decreased GFR, but the degree of metabolic acidosis and hyperkalaemia is far greater than one would expect from the severity of the renal failure. The most severe is Type I renal tubular acidosis. No matter how low the plasma bicarbonate falls, the patient with Type I renal tubular acidosis cannot acidify his urine. Type II is less severe. If the plasma bicarbonate falls low enough the filtered load of bicarbonate falls markedly and urine can be acidified by distal mechanisms alone (a urine of pH6 is bicarbonate-free).

Type II (proximal) RTA may be accompanied by other proximal tubular defects. There may be excessive urinary excretion of glucose, phosphate, amino-acids and uric acid.

Bone disease and nephrocalcinosis are commonly associated with Type I (distal) RTA. Increased calcium excretion is commonly associated with Type I RTA, but not Type II because the distal delivery of bicarbonate in a Type II RTA encourages distal calcium reabsorption.

There are two main mechanisms that can be responsible for the Type I distal RTA:

a: The cellular mechanism responsible for hydrogen ion secretion may be defective. This appears to be the commonest mechanism.
b: Back diffusion of hydrogen ions may occur as the tubular cells may not be able to maintain a hydrogen ion gradient across their cell membrane. This mechanism appears to operate in the distal RTA produced by amphotericin toxicity.

For distal acidification to occur there must be sufficient sodium being delivered to the distal nephron, an adequate aldosterone secretion and tubular responsiveness. Adequate distal sodium exchange is essential to prevent excessive electrochemical differences from developing with the secretion of hydrogen ions.

Proximal RTA

Formal testing of the proximal tubule's ability to conserve bicarbonate requires bicarbonate loading and measurement of the tubular maximal reabsorption of bicarbonate ($TmHCO_3^-$). Sodium loading, however, produces volume expansion which inhibits proximal tubular sodium reabsorption. For this reason the more prolonged oral bicarbonate loading is to be preferred to the shorter infusion test but both will be described.

Bicarbonate infusion test

6 a.m.: An oral load of 0.1g/kg body weight of ammonium chloride in gelatine capsules is given to reduce the plasma bicarbonate to less than 20mmol/l. This step may be omitted if the plasma bicarbonate is already less than 20mmol/l.

10 a.m.: An infusion of 5% sodium bicarbonate is set up and administered at a rate that produces a rise in the plasma bicarbonate of 1–1.5mmol/l/hour. Once the urine pH is above 7.5 the rate of bicarbonate infusion is doubled. Plasma bicarbonate should be elevated to at least 30mmol/l.

Hourly blood samples are collected for plasma bicarbonate and creatinine. Hourly urine volumes are collected for creatinine clearance (as an approximation for GFR) and bicarbonate. Alternatively, GFR may be measured by ^{51}Cr EDTA clearance.

Oral bicarbonate loading test:

6 a.m.: Ammonium chloride is given as above if the plasma bicarbonate is above 20mmol/l.

10 a.m.: Arterial blood is obtained by direct puncture for pH and standard bicarbonate. The base deficit is calculated and the amount of bicarbonate needed to elevate the plasma bicarbonate to 30mmol/l is obtained from the following:

$$(30\text{-}measured\ plasma\ HCO_3{}^-) \times Body\ Weight \times 0.6$$

Half the calculated dose of bicarbonate is then given as sodium bicarbonate capsules.

Regular hourly urine volumes are collected and the plasma bicarbonate and creatinine checked every hour.

Every 15 minutes a further 2g of sodium bicarbonate is given.

Calculation of Tm HCO_3^- and HCO_3^- threshold (**79**).

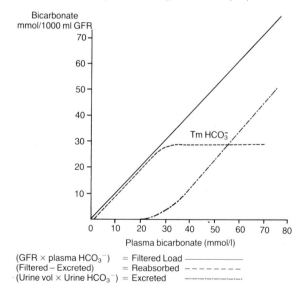

(GFR × plasma $HCO_3{}^-$)	= Filtered Load —————
(Filtered – Excreted)	= Reabsorbed – – – – – – –
(Urine vol × Urine $HCO_3{}^-$)	= Excreted —·—·—·—·—·—

79 Tm Bicarbonate

Interpretation of results: In normal subjects bicarbonate does not appear in the urine until the plasma level is about 26mmol/l (threshold). In a proximal RTA the urine contains bicarbonate when the plasma bicarbonate is below the normal threshold. In a proximal RTA 15% or more of the filtered load of bicarbonate may appear in the urine.

The test may be contraindicated in patients with heart disease and other oedematous states as the sodium load may precipitate heart failure.

Distal RTA – ammonium chloride loading test (short)
The ammonium chloride loading test is often used as a screening test for renal tubular acidosis. It does not indicate whether the lesion is either distal or proximal, unlike the bicarbonate infusion test which is specific for proximal renal tubular acidosis.

Method
8 a.m.:   Baseline blood samples are taken for electrolytes, urea, creatinine and bicarbonate. Two accurately timed hourly urine volume samples are also collected.

10 a.m.:   Oral load of 0.1g/kg body weight of ammonium chloride in gelatine capsules is administered over a period of 60 minutes or less.

Following this, hourly urine volumes are collected for pH, titratable acidity and ammonium estimation over the next six hours. Plasma bicarbonate should be checked every two hours. Arterial blood may be taken for pH at two-hourly intervals to confirm that a systemic acidosis does indeed develop.

Interpretation of results: A normal subject should be able to produce a urine pH of less than 5.3 by four hours after the ammonium chloride load. The maximum rate of total acid excretion should be 40–80mmol per 24 hours. Titratable acidity should be $7–21\mu$mol/min and ammonium excretion $30–50\mu$mol/min. Plasma bicarbonate and chloride should not change by more than 6mmol/l from the initial control period.

The test is only valid if the plasma bicarbonate was reduced to below the threshold of the proximal tubule, i.e. to below 26mmol/l. A normal result excludes a Type I RTA. The fractional excretion of HCO_3^- does not exceed 5% in Type I RTA.

Type IV RTA – prolonged ammonium chloride loading test
In Type IV RTA the kidney can produce an acid urine but cannot maxi-

mally acidify. It is therefore necessary to perform a prolonged ammonium chloride test to reveal this more subtle defect of urinary acidification. The prolonged test stresses the kidney's ability to maximally acidify urine. Unlike other patients with RTA, patients with a Type IV RTA have a marked hyperkalaemia due to the lack of aldosterone secondary to hypo-reninaemia.

Method: A control period of three consecutive days is required during which serial timed 24-hour urine collections are made into bottles containing 10ml liquid paraffin. On the morning of day four 0.1g/kg of ammonium chloride is administered. This is given daily for the next five days. Early morning urine samples on the next six consecutive mornings are tested for pH. Ammonium excretion and titratable acidity should be assayed on the 24-hour urine collections collected after the early morning urine sample has been tested.

Interpretation of results: Normal subjects should reduce their urine pH to 5.0 or less (early morning sample). Ammonium excretion and titratable acidity should increase by $\geqslant 120$mmol/24 hours (approximately 80µmol/min). The plasma bicarbonate should not fall by more than 6mmol/l.

N.B. Ammonium chloride loading tests are contraindicated in liver disease.

Urine – Plasma pCO_2

Rationale: An elegant way of differentiating proximal and distal RTA is to compare the urinary to plasma pCO_2. In a proximal RTA, bicarbonate is not reclaimed and arrives at the distal tubule to meet secreted hydrogen ions.

$$HCO_3^- + H^+ \rightleftharpoons H_2CO_3$$

The distal nephron lacks carbonic anhydrase so the next reaction is delayed and takes place after the urine has left the kidney.

$$H_2CO_3 \rightleftharpoons CO_2 + H_2O$$

Under these circumstances, urinary pCO_2 will rise.

In a distal RTA little or no bicarbonate reaches the distal nephron as it is reclaimed proximally and urine pCO_2 remains low as distal H^+ secretion is defective.

Method: Urine is made maximally alkaline by the intravenous or oral administration of sodium bicarbonate. Plasma bicarbonate should be raised to at least 33mmol/l and a urine pH of greater than 7 should be achieved. This may be done by the administration of intravenous sodium bicarbonate (8.4%) at a rate of 1–2ml/min for two hours. Alternatively, an oral load of 200mmol of sodium bicarbonate can be given the night before the test with overnight water restriction. Urine and blood pCO_2 may be checked at 6 a.m. or, alternatively, half-an-hour after the end of the intravenous infusion of sodium bicarbonate.

Interpretation: Normals: Urine pCO_2 – Blood pCO_2 $\geqslant$30mmHg. Distal RTA: Urine pCO_2 – Blood pCO_2 <15mmHg.

Sodium sulphate test

Rationale: Sulphate ions are not reabsorbed. On arrival at the distal tubule they provide a steep electro-chemical gradient which encourages the maximal secretion of hydrogen ions. If a mineralocorticoid is also administered, this further increases distal hydrogen ion excretion.

Method: Patients should be on a low salt diet for three days. At 12 mid-night and 6 a.m. the following morning, 0.5–1mg of 9-alpha-flurohydro-corticosterone (Fludrocortisone) is administered. At 12 midday, 0.5–1 litre of 4% sodium sulphate is infused over 40–60 minutes. Hourly urine volumes are collected for four hours after the end of the intravenous infusion and tested for pH.

Interpretation: The normal subject should reduce the urine pH to less than 5.3. Most subjects can actually reduce the urine pH to less than 5.0.
   This test resolves several possible causes of impaired distal acidification.

1. By giving non-reabsorbable sulphate anions it ensures an adequate negative intratubular potential and delivery of sodium to the distal tubule. This is important as dehydration and sodium depletion per se impair distal acidification.
2. It can distinguish between the two common causes of impaired distal acidification:

   a: Increased passive back diffusion of hydrogen ions in the distal tubules: sulphate ions trap hydrogen ions in the distal tubule and prevent back diffusion.
   b: Impaired secretion of hydrogen ions: the presence of sulphate ions in the tubular lumen will not correct a basic cellular defect in hydrogen ion secretion.

Calcium chloride test

Patients who are unable to tolerate an oral load of ammonium chloride may be given calcium chloride instead. This also has the advantage that it may be safely used in patients with liver disease.

Rationale: Oral calcium chloride causes the loss of bicarbonate ions in the stool because of the following reaction which occurs in the small bowel:

$$2Na\ HCO_3 + Ca\ Cl_2 \rightleftharpoons Ca\ CO_3 + 2Na\ Cl + CO_2 + H_2O.$$

Method: An oral dose of 1mmol/kg (2mEq/kg) body weight of calcium chloride dissolved in water is administered. Urine samples are tested hourly for the next eight hours.

Interpretation of results: Normal subjects should reduce urine pH to <5.3.

Assays used for the assessment of urinary acidification

Urine that is being tested for pH, bicarbonate and ammonium should be collected under paraffin (or taken into a syringe which is then capped until assayed) to prevent the loss of carbon dioxide.

Urine pH: pH indicator papers are not sufficiently accurate for formal testing of the kidneys' ability to produce an acid urine. pH should be measured using a glass electrode.

Ammonium: Urinary excretion of ammonium is measured by utilising the Berthelot reaction (phenol-hypochlorite), which produces a blue colour.

Bicarbonate: A Titrimetric method can measure bicarbonate directly or a gasometric method can be used which measures carbon dioxide liberated after the addition of acid.

Titratable acidity: 0.1N sodium hydroxide is added to urine to back titrate the pH to 7.4.

Urine pCO_2: Membrane electrodes measure pCO_2 directly.

Tests of proximal tubular function

Tubular reabsorption of glucose

Tubular handling of glucose: Glucose is normally completely reabsorbed by the proximal tubule, so that normal glucose excretion in the urine is less than 5–6mmol/24 hours (100mg/24 hours).

$$Filtered\ load\ of\ glucose = GFR \times Plasma\ concentration$$
$$= 90mg/min\ (0.5mmol/min).$$

There is an upper limit for tubular reabsorption of glucose, so that once the plasma glucose level rises above 10mmol/l (180mg/dl) glucose will appear in the urine. This filtered load at which glucose first appears in the urine is referred to as the renal threshold. The maximum rate of tubular reabsorption of glucose is referred to as the TmG or tubular maximal reabsorption of glucose. It can be seen that the normal filtered load of glucose is well below the TmG.

TmG is a good index of the total functional capacity of the proximal tubule.

Normal values (corrected for $1.73M^2$ body surface area):

$$TmG\ males\quad 375 \pm 80\ mg/min\ (2.1 \pm 0.4mmol/min)$$
$$females\ 303 \pm 55\ mg/min\ (1.7 \pm 0.3mmol/min)$$

Renal plasma threshold:

$$by\ extrapolation:\quad 300mg/dl.\ (16mmol/l)$$
$$actual\ ('splay'):\quad 180mg/dl\ (10mmol/l)$$

Estimation of TmG

Method: A glucose infusion of 20–50% dextrose is set up. To prevent damage to peripheral veins a long catheter is needed, ending in a large central vein. The intravenous rate is adjusted to produce a slow rise in the plasma glucose. During the infusion period liberal oral water is given to ensure an adequate urine output. Half-hourly blood samples are taken for plasma glucose and creatinine. Half-hourly complete urine volumes are collected and assayed for glucose and creatinine. Blood glucose should be raised to about 45mmol/l (800mg/dl) for at least one hour. For each collection period the following calculations are made:

1. Filtered load of glucose = GFR × plasma glucose.
2. Excreted glucose = urine volume × urine glucose concentration.
3. Absorption rate = filtered load – excreted load.

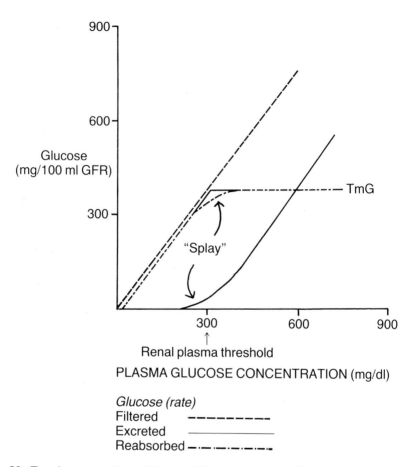

80 Tm glucose and renal threshold for glucose excretion

For accurate studies ^{51}Cr EDTA clearance should be used to measure GFR rather than relying on a creatinine clearance. The patient should be encouraged to drink liberally so that the urine flow rate is fast. Inability to provide accurate and complete urine samples on demand will make this test unreliable. For day-to-day clinical practice it is clearly unsuitable to catheterise patients just to obtain accurate urine volumes.

Interpretation of results: Not all nephrons have the same TmG so there is a degree of splay on the graph, as shown in **80**. TmG is affected by GFR and the extra-cellular fluid volume. Glucose handling is linked to sodium transport so that under conditions of augmented sodium transport glucose transport also increases and the TmG rises.

The test is cumbersome and time-consuming and is more of an interest to physiologists than to clinicians.

For practical purposes the presence of glucose in the urine is always abnormal. It may be due to reduced tubular reabsorption, in which case the plasma glucose will be normal or even low. It may, alternatively, be due to an excessive filtered load, in which case the plasma glucose will be high (diabetes mellitus).

Phosphate reabsorption

Phosphate is normally almost completely reabsorbed by the proximal tubule, with only 10–20% of the filtered load appearing in the urine. The main factor controlling phosphate reabsorption is parathyroid hormone (PTH), which acts on the proximal tubular cells to inhibit phosphate reabsorption. Most of the phosphate handling occurs in the proximal tubule, with only 30% or so being reabsorbed more distally. There are several available indices of renal phosphate handling which can be used clinically.

Theoretical renal phosphorus threshold (TRPT): Stamp and Stacey (see reference) have developed a simple infusion technique to measure the theoretical renal phosphorus threshold (TRPT). As the renal phosphorus threshold is the plasma concentration of phosphorus at which phosphorus first appears in the urine, then

$$GFR \times TRPT = TmP$$

where

GFR = *glomerular filtration rate*
$TRPT$ = *theoretical renal phosphorus threshold*
TmP = *tubular maximal reabsorptive capacity for phosphate.*

Method: The patient fasts overnight:

9 a.m.:   2–3 litres of water are given orally spread over three hours to ensure a good flow of urine. Blood samples are taken every 15 minutes and careful, accurately timed 30-minute urine collections are made starting at 10 a.m.

10 a.m.:   Patient voids and the urine is discarded.

10–10.30 a.m.: First 30-minute urine collection – control period.
10.30–11 a.m.: Second 30-minute urine collection – control period.
11 a.m.:   Infusion set up.
        Fluid: 0.1 molar sodium phosphate (pH 7.4).
        ($Na_2 HPO_4.2H_2O$ 13.8g; $NaH_2 PO_4.2H_2O$ 3.6g plus water to
        1 litre final volume.)

Infusion rate: A pump is required and should be calibrated prior to carrying out the test.

Initial infusion rate:	0.5–1ml/min.
Final infusion rate:	5–10ml/min.

In adults with a normal GFR the higher rates are used. In small subjects and subjects with renal impairment (reduced GFR) less phosphate is required.

The infusion rate is increased by equal increments every 15 minutes over a three-hour period (12 increments) to produce the maximal infusion rate at three hours. This produces a linear rise in plasma phosphate which should not exceed 10mg/dl.

TRPT can be estimated by extrapolating the graph of urine phosphate excretion (mmol or mg/min) against plasma phosphate (same units) to zero.

Normal Values:

TRPT (adults) = 2.7–4.1mg/dl.
= 0.87–1.32mmol/l

In primary hyperparathyroidism, osteomalacia and proximal tubular lesions TRPT is reduced. In patients with hypoparathyroidism or pseudo-hypoparathyroidism, TRPT will be increased.

Errors: Inability to void on demand will invalidate the test. In patients with a marked reduction in GFR the test becomes unreliable.

Maximum tubular reabsorptive capacity for phosphate (TmP): The phosphate infusion test as described above can be used to calculate TmP as described for TmG.

Normal values:

$3.84 \pm 0.84mg/min/1.73m^2$
$124 \pm 27\mu mol/min/1.73m^2$

Tubular reabsorption of phosphate (TRP): Phosphate clearance can be expressed as a ratio of GFR or creatinine clearance to give an index of renal tubular handling of phosphate.

$$TRP = 1 - \frac{(Phosphate\ clearance)}{(GFR\ or\ creatinine\ clearance)} \times 100$$

thus, using creatinine clearance:

$$TRP = 1 - \frac{(Up \times Pc)}{(Pp \times Uc)} \times 100$$

where

Up = Urine concentration of phosphate
Pp = Plasma concentration of phosphate
Uc = Urine concentration of creatinine
Pc = Plasma concentration of creatinine.

Since there is a ratio of clearances, urine volumes cancel out. The test can therefore be performed on an early morning specimen of urine.

Normal value: $>85\%$

Interpretation of results: Excessive urine losses of phosphate can occur in proximal tubular diseases such as the Fanconi syndrome, and may also be seen in primary or secondary hyperparathyroidism. So many other factors affect renal handling of phosphate that formal measurement of TmP is seldom carried out. For most clinical purposes TRP is usually adequate. A nomogram for the estimation of TmP/GFR from simultaneous measurements of TRP and plasma phosphate is available from Bijvoet's studies.

Urinary amino-acid excretion

Tubular transport of amino-acids: There are probably four main groups of amino-acid transport systems in the proximal tubule:

1. Mono-amino-monocarboxylic acids
2. Dibasic
3. Dicarboxylic
4. Imino.

It is thought that a specific intracellular transport protein is responsible for each of these four groups.

Evaluation: Urine can be readily examined by thin layer chromatography to demonstrate the presence or absence of amino-acids in the urine. In the Fanconi syndrome, amino-acids from all four groups are present. In cystinuria, dibasic acids are found in increased amounts. In Hartnup disease, the mono-amino and mono-carboxylic acids are present in increased amounts in the urine.

Cystinuria and monocystinuria: The cyanide-nitroprusside test detects cystine and homocystine and should be carried out as a screening test in selected patients with renal calculi.

Tubular secretion

Sodium para-amminohippurate (PAH) is filtered freely at the glomerulus and secreted by the proximal tubule. At low plasma concentrations (<5mg/dl) the clearance of PAH measures renal plasma flow (Chapter 3, p. 74). If high plasma concentrations are produced (≥20mg/dl) then the active tubular transport mechanism will be saturated. Under these conditions:

PAH excretion = Urine volume × UPAH
PAH filtered = GFR × Plasma concentration
Maximal PAH secretion = (PAH excretion) – (PAH filtered)

GFR should be measured by ^{51}Cr EDTA clearance for accurate results.
Normal values:

Males $80 \pm 17mg/min$
Females $77 \pm 11mg/min.$

The test is more of interest to physiologists and has been used in clinical research rather than routine medical practice.

Lithium Clearance

Recent studies have suggested that lithium is exclusively reabsorbed in the proximal tubule in parallel with sodium and water. No lithium is secreted or reabsorbed in the distal tubules. Therefore changes in lithium clearance reflect changes in proximal tubular function. The clearance of lithium should equal the rate of delivery of sodium and water into the thin descending limb of the loop of Henlé. Measurement of lithium clearance is carried out after the oral ingestion of a single dose of lithium carbonate (10mg/kg body wt) the night before urine is collected. The single oral dose gives a steady plasma level of lithium of about 0.2 to 0.5mmol/l (approximately half the therapeutic blood level) sufficient for an accurate 7 hour urine collection period. Serum lithium is measured by flame photometry; (plasma obtained from blood collected into lithium heparin tubes obviously cannot be used). Patients should take plenty of fluid.

Normal values: 20 ± 2ml/min

Results can also be expressed at a ratio of lithium clearance to creatinine clearance (Normal values: 0.19 ± 0.02)

Lithium excretion rises with increased sodium excretion so that patients should be on a defined sodium intake if results are to be comparable. It is important that a high urine flow rate is obtained – urine should be maximally dilute.

Distal chloride handling

In patients with suspected Bartter's Syndrome it is helpful to assess the distal (loop of Henlé) reabsorption of chloride. Patients with severe hypochloraemic metabolic alkalosis and chloride in the urine may have excessive urinary losses (e.g. diuretics or Bartter's Syndrome). Very low urinary chloride occurs after excessive losses of gastric secretions (e.g. vomiting or naso-gastric aspiration) and in Chloridorrhoea in which the faecal loss of chloride is excessive.

Principle

An indirect assessment of chloride handling by the ascending limb of the loop of Henlé may be obtained as follows:

Free water is generated by the ascending limb of the loop of Henlé by the reabsorption of chloride without water and therefore:

Distal chloride reabsorption = Free water clearance.

The amount of chloride delivered to the ascending limb of the loop of Henlé may be approximated:

Distal chloride delivery = distal chloride reabsorption + chloride excretion.

Fractional distal chloride reabsorption =

$$\frac{Free\ water\ clearance}{Free\ water\ clearance\ +\ chloride\ clearance}$$

Results

Bartter's Syndrome = <0.5 (NB also loop diuretics)
Loss of GI tract secretions = >0.8

6: SPECIALISED INVESTIGATIONS: BIOPSIES AND ENDOSCOPIES

Renal biopsy

Precautions

a: It is important that the patient should be co-operative and capable of holding his breath for at least half a minute. He should be able to obey simple commands to control his breathing.

b: Coagulation and clotting studies should be normal:
> Platelet count
> Prothrombin time
> Partial thromboplastin time
> Thrombin time.

If there is any doubt about a risk of bleeding, a formal bleeding time should be carried out, particularly if the patient is in renal failure.

c: For a percutaneous biopsy, the patient should have two normal-sized kidneys. Open biopsy is indicated for the patient with a single kidney, unless this is a renal transplant kidney.

d: Blood pressure should be normal.

e: Sterile urine

f: Haemoglobin should be more than 8g/dl in case haemorrhage follows the biopsy.

g: Renal function should be such that the loss of one kidney would not mean that immediate dialysis is necessary. This usually means that the patient will have kidneys of normal size, and that the plasma creatinine will be below 300µmol/l. In acute nephritis and acute renal failure, the creatinine may well be much higher than this, but a biopsy may still need to be carried out. The purpose of this particular precaution and the strictures about the size of the patient's kidneys is to prevent attempts at renal biopsy in a patient with unequivocal chronic disease. Such biopsies are difficult and dangerous. They are also not informative. An end-stage kidney looks similar histologically whatever the initial disease. A closed renal biopsy is contraindicated in the following:

Cysts	Macroscopic variety of PAN
Tumours	Perinephric abscesses
Hydronephrosis	Acute pyelonephritis.

Method

The technique needs to be demonstrated and supervised by an experienced practitioner. Briefly, the kidney may be located in one of three ways:

a: From the IVU film and surface markings.
b: By ultrasound immediately prior to the biopsy.
c: Under X-ray screening at the time of the biopsy. This last method is preferable.

The biopsy is taken from the middle of the lower pole of the left kidney, on full inspiration. The left side is to be preferred to avoid the risk of trauma to the liver. Full aseptic precautions and generous local anaesthetic are required. If a second biopsy is necessary, it should be taken from the contra-lateral kidney to reduce the risk of hitting the previous scar or of hitting an arterio-venous fistula that may have been produced from the first biopsy. After a biopsy, 24 hours' complete bed rest is usually advised.

Two cores should be taken, using a Tru-cut℗ or a Franklin modified Vim-Silverman needle. To ensure an adequate specimen, it is helpful to have an assistant identify glomeruli with a dissecting microscope at the time of the biopsy. If an insufficient or inadequate core has been obtained, a further attempt may be made. To maximise the information that can be obtained from a renal biopsy, at least three separate techniques need to be carried out:

a: Light microscopy with special stains (fibrin, amyloid, basement membrane).
b: Electron microscopy.
c: Immunofluorescence with stains for IgG, IgM, IgA, C3 and fibrinogen. Specific deposits of immune reactants can also be revealed by the immunoperoxidase technique.

Complications

Bleeding is the most serious and most common complication after renal biopsy. It is usually produced as a result of one of the following problems:

a: The biopsy site is too high and too medial. One aims to be in the sagittal line that is just lateral to the outermost calyx. The biopsy needle must also be inserted exactly perpendicular to the skin surface of the patient, otherwise surface markings become meaningless.
b: In a small adult or child, the biopsy may be too deep as well as too medial.
c: Holding the needle when the patient is breathing can tear the kidney.

d: Poor positioning of the patient.

e: Attempts to biopsy a patient with chronic renal failure.

f: Uncontrolled hypertension.

g: Lack of patient co-operation or movement during the procedure.

Once bleeding has occurred, adequate replacement of blood is mandatory. The blood pressure should be controlled, if this is not already being done, and it is worth rechecking the clotting studies, including a bleeding time. Bed rest is essential. If bleeding is profuse, an attempt should be made to embolise the bleeding point by selective renal arteriography. This technique is often effective, and may save the patient from emergency nephrectomy (see **49**).

Indications
The principal indications for a renal biopsy are listed in Table 28. Ideally, the biopsyist should be convinced that the result will alter his management before he exposes the patient to the (admittedly small) risk and discomfort of a renal biopsy.

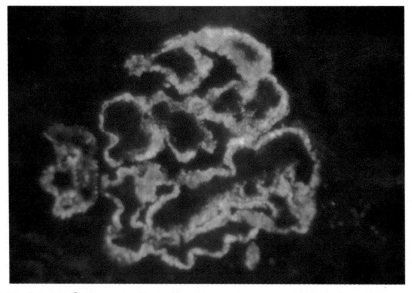

81 Immunofluorescence: Granular pattern. Frozen section (6μ) of renal tissue stained with FITC labelled sheep anti-human IgG. Heavy granular peripheral capillary loop deposits of human IgG have been demonstrated. This appearance is typical of membranous glomerulonephritis (× 300).

Table 28: Indications for renal biopsy

Nephrotic Syndrome
Nephritic Syndrome
Unexplained acute renal failure
Asymptomatic proteinuria
Unexplained haematuria

Interpretation of results

Detailed descriptions of renal pathology are beyond the scope of this book. A properly examined renal biopsy will answer the following questions:

a: Is the disease immunologically mediated? Immunofluorescence or immunoperoxidase studies may demonstrate the deposition of immune reactants (immunoglobulin and complement) in the glomeruli, and less commonly around the tubules. If the deposits are granular

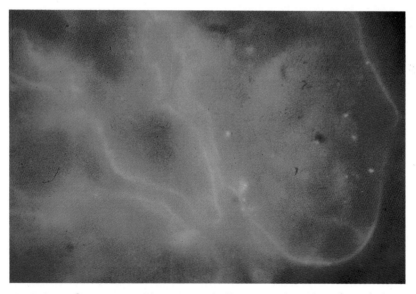

82 Immunofluorescence: Linear pattern. Frozen section (6μ) of renal tissue stained with FITC labelled sheep anti-human IgG (× 2,000). A continuous linear deposit of human IgG along the glomerular basement membrane is shown. This appearance is typical of anti-GBM anti-body mediated glomerulonephritis.

along the glomerular basement membrane (81), this implies an immune complex mediated disease process. Presumptive immune deposits may also be demonstrated by electron microscopy, e.g. SLE (83). A linear deposition of immunoglobulin along the glomerular basement membrane (82) implies that the disease is due to an auto-antibody against glomerular basement membrane antigens. Allergic interstitial nephritis may also be diagnosed on biopsy by the demonstration of an intense peri-tubular and interstitial inflammatory cell exudate, containing mononuclear cells and eosinophils (84).

b: Will the lesion respond to treatment with steroids and/or immunosuppressive agents? The minimal change lesion by definition and some mild cases of focal proliferative glomerular nephritis respond to steroids alone. More aggressive lesions, such as focal necrosis (86) with or without crescents, can be controlled with a combination of immunosuppressive treatment, sometimes including plasma exchange. Most other lesions do not respond to immunosuppression.

In acute renal failure most cases do not need a renal biopsy as the lesion is usually ATN (86). However, if doubt as to the diagnosis exists, then a renal biopsy may well be required. Lesions such as acute glomerulonephritis or an acute allergic tubulo-interstitial nephritis may be found and require specific treatment.

c: What is the prognosis? Certain lesions are untreatable and usually progress to end-stage chronic renal failure over a period of four or five years. It is helpful to know this in advance, so that potentially dangerous treatment can be avoided and a realistic plan for renal replacement therapy can be made for the patient. Examples of lesions of this sort include focal segmental glomerulosclerosis, mesangiocapillary glomerulonephritis, diabetes mellitus and advanced amyloidosis. Marked scarring and sclerosis of glomeruli, with tubular atrophy, are depressing findings and suggest that recovery will, at best, be very limited.

Bladder biopsy

A bladder biopsy taken at cystoscopy can be helpful in the diagnosis of tuberculosis, schistosomiasis and tumours.

Prostatic biopsy

A transrectal needle biopsy of the prostate can differentiate the benign prostatic hypertrophy from carcinoma of the prostate.

Ureteric biopsy

Flexible ureteroscopes have recently been introduced. It is now possible to biopsy suspicious lesions in the ureters and even as high as the renal pelvis and calyces.

Endoscopy

Urethroscopy and cystoscopy are important techniques in the investigation of urinary tract disease. Their main role is to identify the cause and the site of lower urinary tract haemorrhage. Suspicious areas in the bladder may be biopsied. Blood may sometimes be seen coming from a particular ureteric orifice, thus lateralising the source of bleeding and allowing subsequent investigations to focus on the appropriate ureter or kidney. At the time of endoscopy it is usual to carry out a careful bimanual pelvic examination to exclude serious pelvic pathology. The examination is greatly facilitated by having the patient fully relaxed under a general anaesthetic.

Divided renal function studies using ureteric catheters have largely been replaced by isotope scanning techniques. Occasionally it is helpful to culture urine from each ureter to lateralise the site of infection or, if haematuria is the problem, to lateralise the source of the blood.

Flexible ureteroscopes enable the ureter and renal pelvis to be visualised. Biopsies or brushings for cytology may be taken from suspicious lesions.

Such are the recent advances in endoscopy that various therapeutic measures can be carried out during the procedure. Stones can be snared, broken or removed. A variety or ureteric stents can be inserted to bypass obstruction. Clot or urate crystals (the tumour lysis syndrome) can be washed out. Endoscopic resection of hypertrophied prostatic tissue and bladder tumours has been routine practice for many years. Nephroscopes have been developed for diagnostic and therapeutic use via direct percutaneous insertion into the kidney.

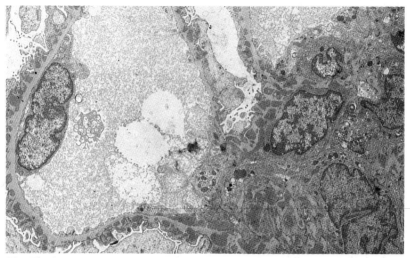

83 Electron microscopy: SLE – electron dense deposits (× 7,500). Two glomerular capillary loops and the mesangial area are shown with extensive subepithelial electron dense deposits around the peripheral capillary loop and in the mesangial area. The deposits are seen to be encroaching upon the subendothelial space. Electron dense deposits on both sides of the basement membrane and in the mesangial area are typical of SLE. There is also mesangial cell proliferation and matrix increase.

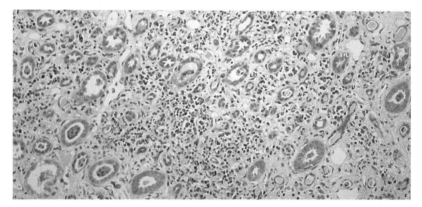

84 Light microscopy: Allergic tubulo-interstitial nephritis (× 150). A renal biopsy (H and E) showing acute tubulo-interstitial nephritis with numerous eosinophils in the spaces around the tubules. This was caused by an allergic reaction to a non-steroidal anti-inflammatory agent.

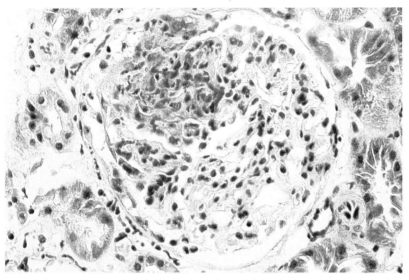

85 Light microscopy: Focal, necrotising glomerulonephritis (× 500 MSB). This is a renal biopsy from a patient with an acute nephritic illness, stained with a trichrome stain. The left half of the glomerulus shows an area of focal necrosis with occasional flecks of fibrin (red). The right half of the glomerulus is relatively normal.

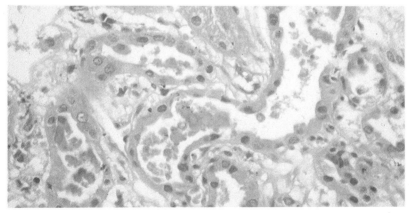

86 Light microscopy: Rhabdomyolysis – ATN (× 600 H & E). This is a renal biopsy from a patient with acute renal failure, stained with haematoxylin and eosin. Tubular damage (ATN) and intratubular myoglobin casts ('brown sugar casts') typical of acute rhabdomyolysis are visible.

7: SPECIALISED INVESTIGATIONS: THE MULTISYSTEM DISEASES

The clinical presentation

The kidney may be involved as part of a multisystem disease. The disease processes may be one of those associated with a diffuse vasculitis or may have a more metabolic 'flavour' (Table 29). A careful history and examination usually points to the correct diagnosis and enables further investigations to be chosen. In some of these diseases the renal involvement can dominate the clinical picture, so that the true multisystem nature of the disease can easily be missed. This is particularly true in cases of systemic lupus erythematosus (SLE) and polyarteritis (87–89).

In general, patients with these diseases will present with one of the following main syndromes:

a: Nephrotic syndrome
b: Nephritic syndrome
c: Acute renal failure.

Investigations

The diagnosis is sometimes obvious but often not, and the patient usually comes to renal biopsy. For many years now it has been the practice of several renal units to carry out a 'biopsy screen', consisting of special tests which ensure that the diagnosis of these multisystem diseases is not missed and that valuable time is not wasted. While it is not always necessary to do all the tests listed in Table 30 in all patients who come to renal biopsy, most are usually indicated. The cost is small with respect to even one day of hospital in-patient care.

Renal function: The basic renal function tests have already been discussed. They serve to demonstrate kidney size, to exclude obstruction and to document renal function. Microscopy of the urine deposit will often provide evidence of parenchymal involvement of the kidney.

Immunology: Immunological assessment ensures that systemic lupus erythematosus is not missed and that more subtle complement deficiencies are also picked up (total complement haemolytic assay – CH50). SLE is diagnosed from the full clinical and laboratory picture. The immuno-fluorescent anti-nuclear factor (ANF) test is a sensitive screening test. The detection and quantitation of antibodies to native double-strand DNA is

Table 29: Multisystem diseases with renal involvement

1	Vasculitides:	Systemic Lupus Erythematosus (SLE)
		Polyarteritis
		Churg-Strauss Syndrome
		Subacute Bacterial Endocarditis (SBE)
		Henoch-Schönlein Purpura (HSP)
		Wegener's Granulomatosis
		Shunt Nephritis
		Goodpasture's Syndrome
2	Metabolic:	Diabetes Mellitus
		Amyloidosis (AA)
		Oxalosis
		Gout
3	Paraproteinaemias:	Multiple Myeloma:
		Hypercalcaemia
		Tubular obstruction
		Amyloidosis (AL)
		Infiltration
		Waldenstrom's Macroglobulinaemia
		Kappa Chain Disease
		Cryoglobulinaemia
4	Haematological:	Sickle Cell Trait/Disease
		Intravascular Coagulation:
		Accelerated Phase Hypertension
		Haemolytic Uraemic Syndrome (HUS)
		Thrombotic Thrombocytopenic Purpura (TTP)
		Toxaemia of Pregnancy
5	Infections:	Streptococcus* ⎫
		Staphylococcus* ⎬ Glomerulonephritis
		Malaria ⎪
		Hepatitis B ⎭
		Leptospirosis ⎫
		Tuberculosis ⎬ Interstitial nephritis

*May also cause ATN from septic shock.

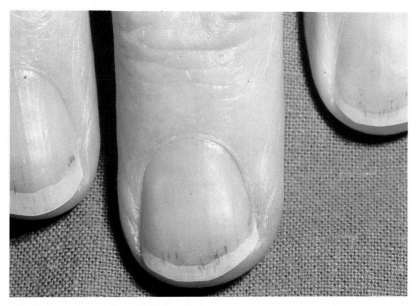

87 Polyarteritis: Splinter haemorrhages

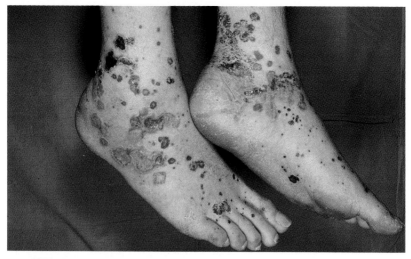

88 HSP: Purpura and necrotic ulcers

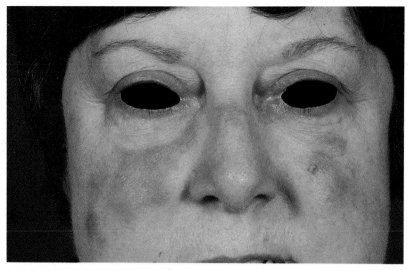

89   SLE: Butterfly rash

confirmatory and of value in monitoring the disease activity in SLE. In addition to SLE there are other diseases affecting the kidney in which complement components may also be depressed (Table 31). A small group of patients with profoundly low C_3 levels and mesangiocapillary glomerulonephritis on a biopsy have been identified as a special group. They have a circulating auto-antibody that permits continued activation of the alternative pathway of complement activation. Tests are available to demonstrate this auto-antibody, which is known as C_3 nephritic factor or C_3 Nef.

Associations between other auto-immune diseases and renal lesions will be identified. For example, membranous glomerulonephritis may complicate thyroid disease. Tubular defects are found in patients with Sjögren's syndrome and in chronic liver disease.

There are numerous tests available for the detection of circulating immune complexes. None is entirely satisfactory, and their impact on clinical management has not been great. They do seem to be of value in monitoring the activity of SLE. A few centres (e.g. Hammersmith Hospital, London) offer a sensitive radio-immunoassay for the detection of the auto-antibodies to glomerular basement membrane.

Recently IgG antibodies to cytoplasmic antigens in polymorphonuclear leucocytes have been detected in patients with Wegener's granulomatosis. Titres may aid diagnosis and indicate the activity of the disease and also polyarteritis.

157

Table 30: The Biopsy Screen

1	Renal:	Urine dip sticks
		Urine microscopy
		Plasma urea, electrolytes and creatinine
		24-Hour urine for creatinine clearance and total protein
		Urine protein selectivity
		MSU for culture
		IVU
		Renal biopsy
2	Immunological assessment:	Complement studies: CH50
		C3
		C4
		Immune complexes
		Anti-glomerular basement membrane and antipolymorph antibodies
		Plasma immunoglobulin levels: IgG, IgM, IgA
		Plasma protein electrophoresis
		Urine protein electrophoresis
		Rheumatoid factor
		Auto-antibodies:
		Thyroglobulin and microsomal antibodies
		Nuclear antibodies
		Smooth muscle antibodies
		Mitochondrial antibodies
		DNA Binding (antibodies to native double strand DNA)
		Cryoglobulins
		HLA typing in some cases
3	Microbiology:	Throat swab
		ASO titre
		Hepatitis B surface antigen
		Blood cultures
		Thick film for malarial parasites
		Syphilis serology

4 Biochemistry: Liver function tests:
Bilirubin
Transaminases
Alkaline phosphatase
Total protein
Albumin
Calcium and phosphate
Creatine phosphokinase
Uric acid
Lactate dehydrogenase
Glucose

5 Haematology: Full blood picture:
Differential white count
Platelets
Film examination
Coomb's test
Coagulation studies and tests for
disseminated intravascular coagulation
Haemoglobin electrophoresis
ESR and C-reactive protein

6 Cardio-respiratory: Chest X-ray
ECG
KCO

Microbiology

An increasing variety of infecting organisms has been implicated in the pathogenesis of glomerulonephritis. We have also become aware of the fact that a tubulointerstitial nephritis may complicate infection, either as a direct result of the infecting micro-organism or sometimes as the result of the chemotherapy. It is extremely important that the diagnosis of sub-acute bacterial endocarditis is not missed. The presence of a fever, a heart murmur and nephritis should alert suspicion and call for at least six blood cultures to be taken. Acute post-streptococcal glomerulonephritis still occurs and will be missed without appropriate tests (ASO titre and throat swab). Positive serology for syphilis may reflect underlying syphilis, but it is also seen in the patient with SLE, who may also have the lupus anticoagulant (an antibody to complex lipoprotein antigens involved in coagulation). Sensitive tests for antibodies to cardiolipin are available to detect the lupus anticoagulant.

Table 31: Reduced complement levels in renal disease

Congenital C2 deficiency and rarer deficiencies

SLE

Early phase of acute post-infection glomerulonephritis

SBE

Shunt nephritis

MCGN

Cryoglobulinaemia

Biochemistry

The association between chronic (immunological) liver disease and tubular defects in the kidney has been commented on. By the time diabetes mellitus causes clinically obvious renal disease, it is usually well advanced with a florid retinopathy. This is not always the case, and a formal glucose tolerance test may occasionally be indicated. Enzyme levels are helpful at diagnosing acute cell damage (e.g. acute rhabdomyolysis by creatine phosphokinase, haemolysis from intravascular coagulation by lactate dehydrogenase, hepatitis by transaminases).

The patient with a high total protein, a normal to high plasma calcium and renal failure may have underlying multiple myeloma revealed by plasma protein electrophoresis and immunoglobulin levels. In addition, the plasma uric acid may be inappropriately high for the degree of renal failure.

Haematology

Full coagulation studies are required prior to renal biopsy. Disturbed coagulation from antibodies to coagulation factors may occur in SLE. Although most patients with the nephrotic syndrome are hypercoagulable, some lose excessive amounts of Factor VII in the urine and may have an increased risk of bleeding. In doubtful cases, it is helpful to extend haematological investigations to look for evidence of intravascular coagulation and micro-angiopathic haemolytic anaemia (MAHA). The blood film may be characteristic with burr cells, helmet cells and other red cell fragments (90). The reticulocyte count is high and there may be a marked leucocytosis. Fibrin degradation products are usually present in the plasma and the platelet count and fibrinogen levels are low from consumption in patients with MAHA.

The full blood picture may provide other clues. A very high ESR is typical of the nephrotic syndrome and multiple myeloma. A neutrophil leucocytosis may be seen in active polyarteritis. Thrombocytosis is sometimes found in Wegener's granulomatosis. SLE can present with a pancytopenia or Coomb's positive haemolytic anaemia. It may also present as acute thrombocytopenic purpura.

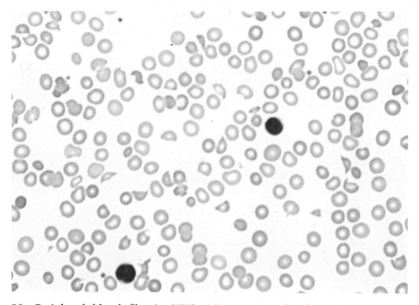

90 Peripheral blood film in HUS: Micro-angiopathic haemolytic anaemia (MAHA) caused by intravascular coagulation in the haemolytic uraemic syndrome (HUS). Note the chopped up erythrocytes and fragments together with sparse platelets. A similar film may be seen in malignant or accelerated phase hypertension and toxaemia of pregnancy.

Cardiorespiratory

The chest X-ray is of value in assessing fluid balance in a renal patient, as well as looking for the nature of the underlying disease. Tuberculosis can be diagnosed from the chest X-ray, but other pneumonias can be associated with glomerulonephritis, e.g. pneumococcal pneumonia. Tubulo-interstitial nephritis may complicate Legionnaire's disease, leptospirosis and tuberculosis. In Goodpasture's syndrome, the X-ray changes range from the subtle to the gross 'white-out' of both lung fields (**91**). Despite a relatively normal radiographic appearance, severe lung haemorrhage may occcur as indicated by a falling haemoglobin. There may be little in the way of frank haemoptysis. This occult lung haemorrhage can be detected by the diffusing capacity for carbon monoxide (KCO) which rises as fresh extravasated blood binds the inhaled carbon monoxide in the lungs. It may be necessary to ventilate the patient, but this can be decided on the basis of arterial blood gases.

The ECG is of value in older patients, those with hypertension and in cases in which a myocarditis can complicate the clinical picture, for example, streptococcal infection, bacterial endocarditis, leptospirosis and SLE, etc.

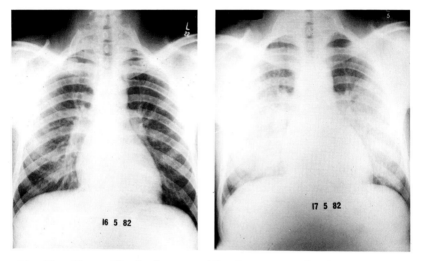

91   Chest X-rays: The development of Goodpasture's syndrome.

8: DIAGNOSTIC PROBLEMS AND CLINICAL SYNDROMES

Haematuria

A positive diagnosis must always be made in the patient with haematuria. Haematuria is always abnormal and may have very serious causes. In the occasional patient in whom a definitive diagnosis is not possible, follow up and repeat investigations may be necessary.

General textbooks of nephrology should be consulted for a classification of causes of haematuria. Suffice it to say here that the major differential diagnosis is between surgical and medical causes (e.g. tumours or nephritis). A careful history and physical examination may indicate the probable cause.

A simplified scheme for investigation of haematuria is given in **92**. It may be possible to eliminate some investigations quickly by a careful assessment of the patient. The age of the patient, the time of the haematuria in relation to urinary stream and the association with pain or dysuria reduces the list of likely causes. Haematuria that persists after infection or control of severe hypertension needs full investigation.

Proteinuria

Nephrologists commonly have to investigate the patient with asymptomatic proteinuria. Routine urine tests are now frequently done for medical examinations at school, university entrance, military service medicals, pre-employment medicals and insurance medicals.

Heavy proteinuria: Proteinuria of more than 2–3g/24 hours usually implies glomerular disease. Patients with severe hypertension, heart failure or constrictive pericarditis can, however, also develop heavy proteinuria. It would be wrong to carry out a full nephrological investigation and a renal biopsy in these patients until hypertension or heart failure has been adequately controlled. If the proteinuria persists, then investigations should proceed along the lines discussed under the heading of 'The Biopsy Screen'.

Asymptomatic proteinuria: Proteinuria under 2g/day is seldom symptomatic. It may be the clue to severe underlying renal disease, especially if accompanied by even slight haematuria. The first thing that has to be done is to confirm the presence of the proteinuria by repeated stick testing on an early morning sample of urine. A positive stick test must be confirmed by a 24-hour urine collection, and accurate quantitation. Intermittent proteinuria is seldom serious. The next test must exclude postural or orthostatic proteinuria (Table 32).

Orthostatic proteinuria

Definition: Proteinuria is present on standing or after ambulation, but disappears during recumbency.

Mechanism: It is thought that the kidney prolapses during upright posture, raising renal venous pressure, which causes the proteinuria.

Test: The patient is instructed to void before retiring at night. Three consecutive early morning urine samples are collected immediately on rising and tested for proteinuria. These are compared with three midday urine samples collected after the patient has been up and about all morning.

Significance: Several long-term studies and renal biopsies have confirmed that the condition is benign. No further action needs to be taken.

If proteinuria is persistent and not orthostatic, then the simple basic tests indicated should be carried out. Thereafter, investigation will follow the outline indicated in **94**.

Table 32: Initial tests for asymptomatic proteinuria

---

1   Confirm: early morning urine dip stick tests × 3
2   Exclude: orthostatic proteinuria
3   Microscopic urine for casts and cells
4   MSU for culture
5   Quantitate 24-hour urine protein excretion
6   Simple renal function tests:
        Plasma urea and creatinine
        24-Hour urine for creatinine clearance

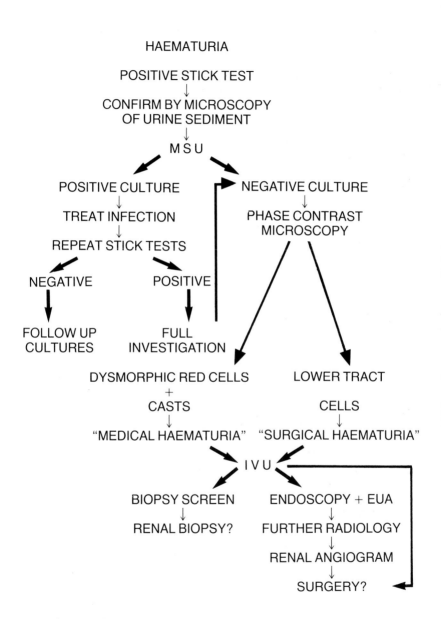

92 Algorithm for the investigation of haematuria.

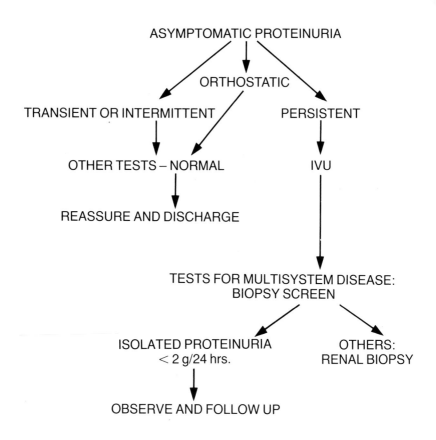

93 Algorithm for the investigation of asymptomatic proteinuria.

Intrarenal mass or space-occupying lesion (SOL)

A plain X-ray, IVU or ultrasound of the kidney may reveal a mass lesion. The main fear is that such a lesion may be a tumour, although there are other possibilities (Table 33).

Careful ultrasound, particularly if combined with cyst puncture, can be diagnostic (**94, 95**). It is worth remembering that simple cysts are common and can co-exist with other unrelated, more serious lesions. The selective renal arteriogram is usually definitive and will demonstrate a pathological circulation in most tumour cases. A note of caution is needed, however, as a few renal tumours are relatively avascular. If a tumour is suspected, the contra-lateral kidney should be checked at arteriography as a proportion of these tumours are bilateral.

Table 33: Differential diagnosis of a suspected intrarenal space-occupying lesion (SOL)

Cyst:
    Single or multiple
    Congenital or acquired
Tumour:
    Benign or malignant
    Primary or secondary
Tumour within the wall of a cyst
Cyst within the centre of a necrotic tumour
Anatomical variants:
    Foetal lobulation
    Dromedary hump (left kidney)
    Cortical islands
    Duplex kidneys
Compensatory hypertrophy
Obstruction
Abscess:
    Tuberculosis
    Hydatid cyst
    Bacterial (diabetics)
Renal sinus fat in the ageing kidney
Trauma
Xanthogranulomatous pyelonephritis
Artefactual:
    Poor quality IVU or ultrasound

Diffuse amorphous calcification related to a solid lesion usually implies a neoplasm (25). Cyst walls, however, do calcify but the calcification does not imply any underlying malignancy. There is still discussion as to whether needle biopsy or aspiration of a solid mass for histology and cytology is safe, or whether it carries an increased risk of disseminating the tumour cells. Some centres now carry out needle aspiration even of solid lesions. Presumed hydatid cysts are not punctured.

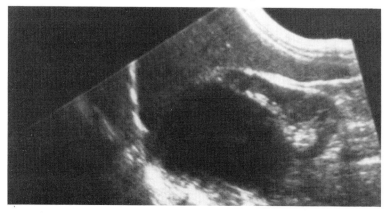

94 Ultrasound: Simple cyst. A large echo free area is seen to the left and inferior to the renal echoes. If doubt exists, cyst can be punctured and contrast introduced to delineate the wall of the cyst.

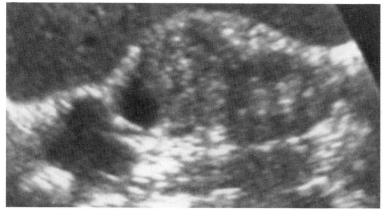

95 Ultrasound: Hypernephroma. There is a solid mass demonstrated in continuity with the kidney which was subsequently shown to be a hypernephroma at nephrectomy. Within the mass lesion is an echo-free area representing a small area of cystic degeneration.

CT scanning is valuable in selected cases to denote perirenal lesions, local tumour spread and retroperitoneal lesions such as lymph nodes. A scheme indicating the approach to investigation of intrarenal lesions is given in **96**.

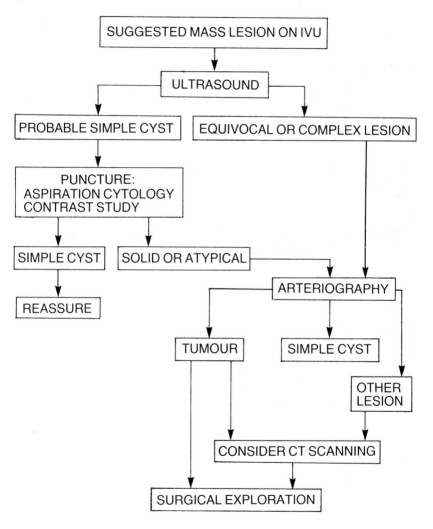

96 Investigation of a renal mass or SOL.

Acute renal failure

The cause of acute renal failure is usually apparent from the clinical context in which it arises. In many cases the aetiology is complex, involving periods of hypotension, sepsis and potentially nephrotoxic antibiotics. There are three important steps that take precedence over the more esoteric investigations:

a: Is the patient in immediate danger from a serious derangement of his biochemistry?
b: Can pre-renal factors be speedily corrected?
c: Has obstruction been excluded?

Immediate danger
Urgent plasma biochemistry to check the plasma potassium and calcium must be requested. Potassium can rise extremely fast in the presence of tissue damage, infection and acute renal failure. Profound hypocalcaemia can occur with hyperkalaemia in acute rhabdomyolysis. Severe hypercalcaemia itself can cause acute renal failure and may culminate in a cardiac arrest. A severe metabolic acidosis with a plasma bicarbonate of less than 10mmol/l is a serious risk to life in itself (with such severe acidoses, lactic acidosis should be considered). Patients who have lost large volumes of upper gastro-intestinal secretions, from vomiting or nasogastric aspiration, can develop acute renal failure. There will be an accompanying profound hypokalaemic, hypochloraemic metabolic alkalosis associated with marked respiratory depression and hypoxia.

Impaired renal perfusion
Special laboratory tests are not usually required to diagnose either cardiac failure or hypovolaemia. Central venous pressure or pulmonary wedge pressure measurement may be needed in difficult cases. Reassurance that the kidney is potentially recoverable with restoration of perfusion can be obtained from analysing the quality of the urine (Table 26, see p. 130). Pre-renal factors must be corrected speedily to prevent the development of established acute tubular necrosis. These criteria relating to the quality of the urine are only valid if the patient is oliguric and not receiving diuretics.

Obstruction
Obstruction can be excluded by either an ultrasound or a high dose IVU. There is now increasing concern that X-ray contrast media may be nephrotoxic although the new non-ionic contrasts appear safe provided dehydration/hypovolaemia is not present. It may be as well to avoid a

high dose IVU in acute renal failure where possible. If an IVU is done, the patient must not be dehydrated. A plain KUB X-ray with tomograms of the renal areas must be taken before giving the contrast. An immediate one-minute film with tomograms taken after the injection of contrast medium will demonstrate renal perfusion. It may be important to continue the study for up to 24 hours if obstruction is to be excluded. In many centres, a careful ultrasound has replaced the emergency high dose IVU in the assessment of acute renal failure. If this approach is chosen then a plain X-ray of the KUB area and renal tomograms should be taken. If there is any doubt about adequate renal perfusion, then an emergency DTPA renogram may be performed as an alternative to an IVU. DSA may have a place in this context when it becomes more widely available. CT scanning (with contrast) is particularly helpful for detecting extrarenal obstruction due to retroperitoneal or pelvic pathology.

Once the early stage of resuscitation-investigation is over, more detailed investigations looking for the cause of acute renal failure may be undertaken. The range of investigations is essentially the same as those that have been discussed under the heading of 'The Biopsy Screen'. A renal biopsy is indicated in acute renal failure for the rare patient who presents with a fulminating crescentic glomerulonephritis or an allergic interstitial nephritis. Most of the patients presenting with acute renal failure will have acute tubular necrosis (ATN) and a renal biopsy will not be indicated.

Later investigations may need to be done if the patient fails to recover from what appeared to be a simple episode of ATN. A plain KUB may show the appearance of cortical calcification if cortical necrosis has developed. Isotope scans, either with DMSA or with DTPA, are helpful and reassure the clinician that perfusion of the kidneys continues and that recovery is still possible. A renal biopsy may be necessary at this late stage, but it carries an extra risk of haemorrhage in the uraemic patient. The purpose of the biopsy at this late stage is to assess whether or not recovery is possible, to ensure that a treatable condition has not been missed (e.g. an underlying glomerulonephritis or an allergic interstitial nephritis from drug therapy).

Glomerulonephritis: Assessment of disease activity

Renal biopsy defines the pattern of injury in the glomerulus and provides evidence for continuing disease activity (e.g. cellular proliferation, infiltration with polymorphs, presence of cellular crescents, foci of necrosis). The biopsy will also document past damage that has healed by fibrosis, leaving glomerular scarring and tubular atrophy.

One difficult problem is how long to continue immunosuppression and

Table 34: Monitoring disease activity

Serial estimations of:
1. Plasma creatinine
2. Creatinine clearance
3. 24-Hour protein excretion
4. Plasma albumin

Serial semi-quantitative assessment of urine deposit:
1. Cells
2. Casts

Non-specific markers of inflammation:
1. ESR
2. C-reactive protein

Immunological markers of active disease, e.g. SLE:
C3
C4
C3 breakdown products
Antibodies to native double-strand DNA
Circulating immune complexes
Titre of antipolymorph antibodies

Assessment of Goodpasture's Syndrome:
Titre of antiglomerular basement membrane antibody
Serial estimation of KCO for lung haemorrhage

Table 35: Factors mimicking disease activity

Development of the nephrotic syndrome:
Intravascular volume depletion producing impaired renal perfusion
Uncontrolled hypertension
Iatrogenic hypotension from anti-hypertensive drugs
Hypovolaemia from excessive use of diuretics
Nephrotoxic drugs
Hypercalcaemia
Drug-induced interstitial nephritis
Hyperperfusion of remaining normal nephrons
Use of non-steroidal anti-inflammatory agents

in what dose once it has been started. If the original disease process has been adequately treated, further immunosuppression is not only useless but potentially hazardous. Careful monitoring of the patient and carefully selected laboratory tests can provide evidence of continuing disease activity. The decision to continue treatment is based on a combination of clinical impression and laboratory investigations (Table 34).

Although the initial acute treatment may have been adequate, renal function can continue to deteriorate for reasons not directly related to the original disease (Table 35). Amongst these is the phenomenon of hyperperfusion of the remaining normal nephrons, which produces progressive scarring and eventual renal failure. This process must be distinguished from activity of the disease, so that unnecessary treatment can be avoided.

Hypertension

The commonest demonstrable cause of hypertension is that of an underlying renal disease. The picture is complicated as hypertension, whatever its cause, will produce renal damage. Almost all renal lesions may produce hypertension by sodium retention and over-activity of the renin-angiotensin system. The evaluation of the hypertensive patient is a common clinical problem for the nephrologist.

It is not necessary to carry out an IVU on every hypertensive patient. However, simple renal function tests should be done, not only to document baseline function but also to look for evidence that the kidney might be the cause of the hypertension (Table 36). An IVU should be carried out if preliminary renal function tests suggest renal impairment. The other investigations to be considered are listed in Table 37.

A renal arteriogram is generally indicated in young patients with severe hypertension and in patients whose hypertension suddenly deteriorates. A helpful test in investigating patients with probable renal artery stenosis is the ^{99m}Tc DTPA renogram before and after a single dose of captopril (25mg). Uptake is reduced on the side of the renal artery stenosis after captopril. This occurs as a consequence of loss of post-glomerular arteriolar tone (Angiotensin II dependent) with the consequent loss of filtration pressure.

Selective renal vein samplings for renin, and comparing renin levels from each kidney with that of the peripheral blood is required to demonstrate a unilateral renal cause for hypertension. A ratio of renal vein renin to systemic venous renin of 1.5 or more suggests that that particular kidney is responsible for the hypertension. Samples may need to be taken from within the kidney from segmental branches of the renal vein. A good response to surgical correction can be expected with

Table 36: Initial investigation of hypertension

Urine	Dip sticks: blood + protein Microscopy if dip sticks positive Culture
Plasma	Urea, Creatinine, electrolytes
ECG	
Chest	X-ray

Table 37: Investigation of hypertension associated with a renal lesion

Initial

24 hour urine: Creatinine clearance
Total protein

Ultrasound and KUB

IVU – rapid sequence films if suspect RAS

^{99m}Tc DTPA renogram – Pre- and post-Captopril if suspect RAS

Subsequent

i Renal biopsy if evidence of bilateral parenchymal disease, eg:
Proteinuria ⎱ persist despite BP control
Haematuria ⎰ (see p. 158, Biopsy screen)

ii If evidence of RAS: (IVU, ^{99m}Tc DTPA renogram)
DSA and Renal vein sampling for renin

^{99m}TC DMSA scan: divided renal function
segmental (intrarenal) stenosis

Bilateral Selective renal arteriogram

iii If evidence of unilateral parenchymal renal disease: ^{99m}TC DMSA scan unilateral high renins. The advent of digital subtraction angiography (DSA) means that the arterial supply of the kidneys can be demonstrated at the time of renal vein sampling for renin.

When unilateral renal disease has been demonstrated, a DMSA scan is helpful to define what proportion of total renal function comes from the diseased kidney. It may prove to be more than was expected and, in the presence of reduced total GFR, should dissuade the surgeon from a hasty nephrectomy in an attempt to cure the hypertension.

In the presence of grade III or grade IV retinopathy (accelerated phase hypertension) tests should be carried out to look for evidence of acute renal damage, excessive production of renin and a micro-angiopathic haemolytic anaemia (MAHA) (Table 38).

As a group the endocrine causes of hypertension are important (Table 39) although individually rather rare. Paroxysmal hypertension and glycosuria may suggest a phaeochromocytoma. Although a low plasma potassium is typical of Conn's and Cushing's Syndrome, it is commonly associated with other states. Any severe hypertension with an elevated renin can produce hypokalaemia. Diuretics are another common cause.

Table 38: Investigation of accelerated phase hypertension

Plasma K$^+$

MAHA: Blood film
         Platelet count

DIC: PT
         PTTK
         FDP

Consider angiography

Monitor renal function carefully: Plasma creatinine
                                     Proteinuria
                                     Creatinine clearance

Table 39: Endocrine related hypertension

Symptoms and signs Initial screening tests	} → possible endocrinopathy?
Phaeocromocytoma:	Urinary VMA Plasma catecholamines Abdominal CT scan ^{131}I Metaiodobenzylguanidine (MIBG) scan
Thyroid disease:	TSH Free T$_4$
Conn's Syndrome:	Urinary K$^+$ ↑ Plasma K$^+$ ↓ Plasma HCO$_3$ ↑ Aldosterone ↑ Renin ↓
Cushing's Syndrome:	Urinary free cortisol ↑
Acromegaly:	Growth hormone Pituitary function tests Skull X-ray

Renal calculi

The nephrologist frequently co-operates with his urological colleagues in screening stone-formers for evidence of an underlying metabolic disorder (Table 40). The morbidity and even mortality from this common disorder requires that every effort is made to prevent further stone formation once the surgeon has effected as good a stone clearance as he is able. Long-term treatment and follow up are also important. The basic screening tests that should be carried out are listed in Table 41. The stone itself should be analysed for the following:

Calcium
Phosphate
Magnesium
Oxalate
Uric acid
Cystine
Xanthine.

Table 40: Metabolic causes of stone formation

Hypercalcuria:
    1   Absorptive hypercalcuria
    2   Hypercalcaemia of any cause
    3   Excretory (renal tubular) hypercalcuria
Hyperuricosuria
Hyperparathyroidism
Cystinuria
Renal tubular acidosis
Oxalosis
Xanthinuria

Table 41: Investigation of stone formers

Stone analysis
Regular urine cultures
Diurnal variation in urine pH
Exclude renal tubular acidosis:
    1 EMU for pH
    2 Ammonium chloride acidification test
24-Hour urine:
    Calcium
    Phosphate
    Oxalate
    Urate and Xanthine
    Magnesium
    Cystine
Fasting plasma:
    Calcium: ionized calcium if available
    Phosphate
    Magnesium
    Urate
    Alkaline phosphatase
    Chloride
    Bicarbonate
Urine $\dfrac{\text{Calcium}}{\text{Creatinine}}$ ratio:
    1 Fasting
    2 After oral calcium load
Tests for hyperparathyroidism:
    1 Plasma PTH
    2 Hand X-rays

Urine amino-acid chromatogram
Screen for cystine

Urine $\dfrac{\text{Calcium}}{\text{Creatinine}}$ ratio

A two hour collection of early morning urine after an over-night fast should be collected and the urine and plasma calcium and creatinine concentrations measured. An oral load of 2.5g of calcium carbonate is given (1.0g of elemental calcium) and a four-hour urine collection is then carried out.

Normal values:

> *Fasting ratio: 0.02–0.16mgca/mg of urinary creatinine*
> *0.06–0.45 mmolca/mmol of urinary creatinine*
> *Post-calcium load ratio = < 0.2 (mgca/mg urinary creatinine)*
> *< 0.57 mmolca/mmol urinary creatinine*

Hypercalcuria is the commonest metabolic abnormality found in stone formers and may result from excessive bone resorption, e.g. hyperparathyroidism, excessive gastrointestinal absorption or a primary renal leak of calcium.

If the difference between the fasting ratio and the ratio after the calcium load is greater than 0.1 (> 0.28 SI units), then the patient has absorptive hypercalcuria. When this is found, measures should be taken to reduce calcium absorption (e.g. diet, sodium cellulose). Thiazide diuretics (not loop diuretics) may be given to reduce urinary calcium excretion.

Assessment of patients in chronic renal failure (CRF)

Most of the foregoing investigations have dealt with the problems of how to measure renal function and how to detect the underlying cause of the renal impairment. Once the diagnosis of CRF has been made and the cause discovered as far as possible, further tests need to be done to assess the complications of uraemia. These may be grouped under the following headings:

a: Cardiovascular system.
b: Haemotology.
c: Musculo-skeletal system.
d: Neurology.
e: Preparation for transplantation.

Cardiovascular system

Pericarditis, complicated by effusion and sometimes tamponade may develop in patients with chronic renal failure. Pericarditis may occur either before or after the onset of dialysis. No specific risk factors have been identified, but the more uraemic the patient the greater the risk appears to be. A chest X-ray will often suggest a pericardial effusion (**97**), but an echocardiogram is diagnostic.

Hypertension is both a cause and a consequence of renal failure, and its effects on the heart should be monitored with ECGs and chest X-rays at regular intervals.

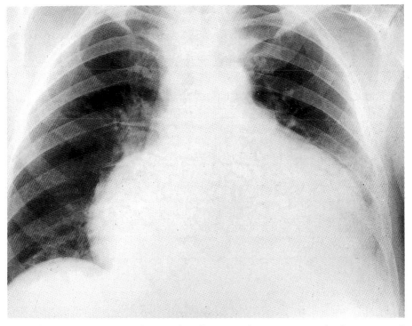

97   Chest X-ray: Pericarditis with effusion. This patient with chronic renal failure has a gross increase in the transverse diameter of the heart, produced by a large pericardial effusion. Note the clear lung fields.

Haematology

The main problem in CRF is that of a refractory normocytic normo-chromic anaemia due for the most part to lack of erythropoietin. The degree of anaemia is related to the severity of the CRF (**98**). Platelets behave abnormally and platelet dysfunction underlies the bleeding tendency in uraemia. Coagulation tests are normal, but the bleeding time may be markedly prolonged, particularly in the presence of certain drugs (Beta-lactam compounds such as penicillins), sepsis or severe uraemia.

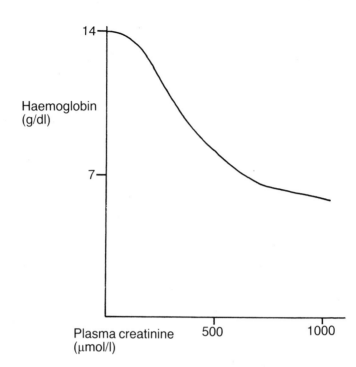

14 —

Haemoglobin
(g/dl)

7 —

Plasma creatinine   500   1000
(μmol/l)

98   Relationship between plasma creatinine and haemoglobin

Musculo-skeletal system

Once GFR falls much below 30%, metabolic bone disease develops
(**99–108**). The best way to assess renal osteodystrophy is by bone biopsy
(**104–106**), but this is invasive and painful. The radiological features
(summarised in Table 42) can be obvious. Dialysis has contributed to the
development of a new bone disease due to aluminium intoxication and its
deposition at the calcification front. Plasma aluminium levels should be
checked regularly in patients with chronic renal failure. The rise in
plasma aluminium after an intravenous dose of 40mg/kg body weight
desferrioxamine can be diagnostic of aluminium intoxication
(> 200μg/l above baseline). A bone biopsy can be carried out and
stained for the presence of aluminium. The regular assessment of renal
osteodystrophy should include the tests listed in Table 43 and may be
repeated annually or more frequently if active treatment is being undertaken.

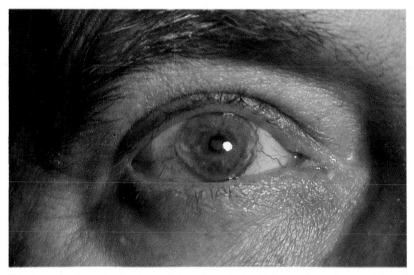

99 Metastatic calcification: Subconjunctival. This patient is at risk of developing the 'red eye of uraemia'. Marked subconjunctival calcification can be seen which in some patients leads to an acute inflammatory reaction. The calcified deposits can be removed by careful scraping under local anaesthetic.

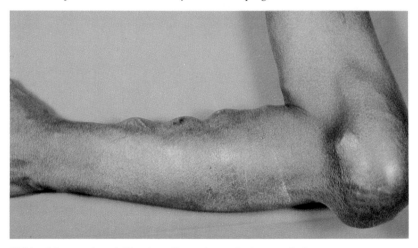

100A Metastatic calcification: Extensive soft tissue calcification can occur in renal failure in patients with marked hyperphosphataemia. This patient developed extensive calcification in the arterio-venous fistula as well as in the bursae around the elbow joints (see **100B**).

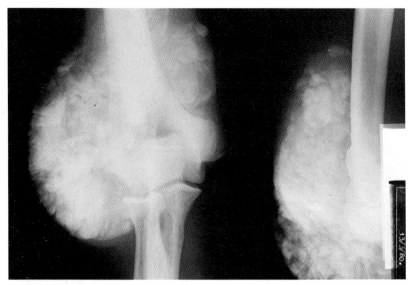

100 B Metastatic calcification. Extensive calcification in the bursae around the elbow joint.

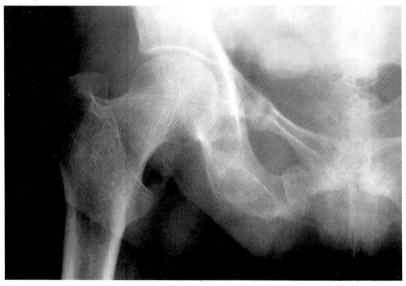

101 Pelvic X-ray: Osteomalacia. A typical Looser's zone is seen here in the superior pubic ramus in a patient with chronic renal failure.

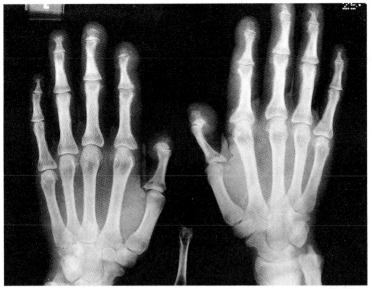

102 Hand X-ray: Hyperparathyroidism. There is marked secondary hyperparathyroidism in this young patient with chronic renal failure. Note the ragged edge to the middle phalanges (sub-periosteal erosions) and the fraying at the ends of the terminal phalanges.

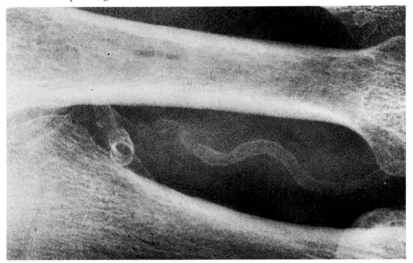

103 Foot X-ray: Vascular calcification. Calcification in the dorsalis pedis artery and interdigital arteries can produce a ring shadow where the vessel is seen end on. (Tatler's sign.)

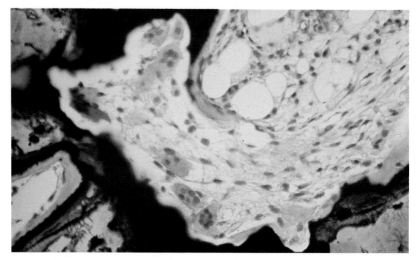

104 Osteitis fibrosa cystica. Multinucleated giant cells (osteoclasts) excavate the mineralized bone to produce a scalloped appearance. The marrow cavity is expanded and extra fibrous tissue is deposited.

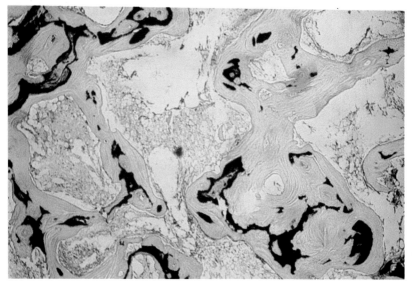

105 Osteomalacia. Mineralized bone (black) is extensively covered by wide seams of osteoid. The marrow cavity is normal.

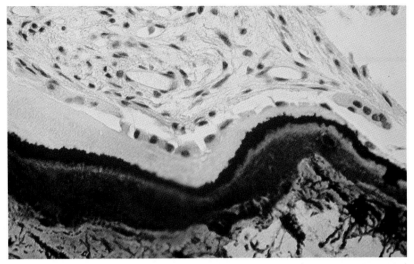

106 **Increased bone turnover.** In patients with renal failure there is increased bone turnover (synthesis + resorption). This section illustrates a row of osteo-blasts lying on the osteoid seam in addition to a multinucleated osteoclast to the right of the field.

Table 42: Radiological features of renal osteodystrophy

Hyperparathyroidism:
  Subperiosteal erosions:
    phalanges
    patella
    lateral ends of clavicles
    neck of femur
    acromion
  Loss of terminal phalanges:
    'tufting'
  Brown tumours

Osteomalacia (adults):
  Pseudo fractures (Looser's zones):
    pubic rami
    ribs
    neck of femur

Renal rickets (children):
  Pelvic deformities
  Ragged epiphyses:
    'champagne cup'
  Long bone deformity:
    genu valgum

Osteoporosis:
  Thin bones:
    decreased mineralisation
    hair-line fractures
    wedging and collapse of vertebral bodies

Osteosclerosis:
  Dense white bones

Aluminium bone disease:
  Fracturing osteomalacia

Metastatic calcification:
  Vessels
  Subconjunctival
  Periarticular

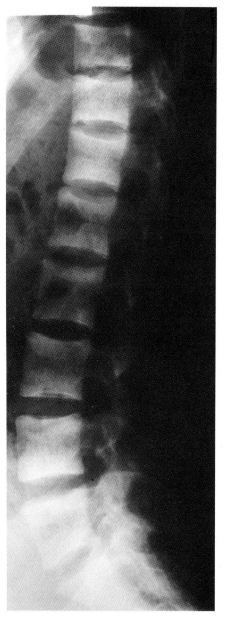

107 Lateral spine X-ray: Osteosclerosis. This lesion produces a 'rugger jersey' spine in patients with chronic renal failure. The appearance is due to alternating bands of sclerosis and rarefaction of the vertebrae.

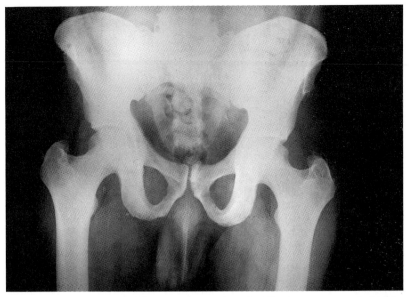

108 X-ray of pelvis and femora: Osteosclerosis. The bone texture is highly abnormal with dense white bones and loss of the usual trabeculae.

Table 43: The assessment of renal osteodystrophy

Plasma:	Fasting calcium and phosphate (ionised calcium where available)
	Albumin
	Alkaline phosphatase (isoenzymes may be required)
	Parathyroid hormone
	Vitamin D metabolites if available
	Aluminium
	Hydroxyproline
Radiology:	Hands
	Spine
	Pelvis
Biopsy:	Selected cases only: Tetracycline labelling
	Aluminium stains

Neurology

With the increasing provision of dialysis facilities, severe uraemic peripheral neuropathy should be relatively infrequent. In a few cases, nerve conduction studies can help by confirming its presence and by monitoring progression after the institution of dialysis therapy. Diabetics require full ophthalmological assessment, with photocoagulation if necessary, before dialysis.

Preparation for transplantation

The patient should have a full urological and nephrological assessment to ensure that he is not only fit enough to undergo a renal transplant but that it is also technically feasible. For a detailed discussion of this topic the reader is referred to textbooks on renal transplantation.

Nephrology: Recently active glomerulonephritis is a relative contraindication to transplantation. If antibodies to glomerular basement membrane can be detected in the serum, the disease will recur in the graft. Most now advise waiting six to twelve months after the last positive antibody test before undertaking a transplant. The multisystem vasculitides should be controlled prior to transplantation.

Immunology: Prior to transplantation full tissue typing (HLA: A, B, C and DR) is carried out. Sera should be screened for the presence of preformed cytotoxic antibodies to HLA antigens and lymphocytotoxic auto-antibodies.

Urological assessment: Urinary tract sepsis (e.g. calculus related) should be eliminated. A micturating cystourethrogram and urodynamic studies may be indicated to ensure that the lower urinary tract is normal and that urinary drainage is adequate.

Microbiology: Active infection is a strong contraindication to transplantation. Foci of infection (teeth, sinuses, lungs etc) can lead to a disseminated infection post-transplantation. Tuberculosis in susceptible groups may be reactivated. CMV antibody status should be checked as most recommend not transplanting a CMV antibody positive donor organ into a CMV antibody negative recipient.

Hepatitis B can produce progressive liver disease after immunosuppression (see below). A pre-transplant eosinophilia should be noted as it can indicate dormant strongyloides infection. With immunosuppression a fatal hyperinfestation syndrome can develop.

Liver disease: Dialysis patients' plasma concentrations of liver transaminases are normally depressed and run at the lower limit of normal.

Normal or slightly elevated levels may mean active liver disease. This is particularly important for patients who carry the hepatitis B virus. Post-transplant, with immunosuppression, progressive liver disease may occur in such patients.

Cardiovascular disease: Peripheral vascular disease is a contraindication to transplantation. Steal syndromes and acclerated atherosclerosis may compromise lower limb circulation (**109**). DSA studies may help to demonstrate the adequacy of the pelvic and lower limb arterial supply. Ischaemic heart disease is also a factor to assess when considering the suitability of a patient for transplantation. Rapid progression of coronary artery disease is common in steroid treated hypertensive transplant recipients.

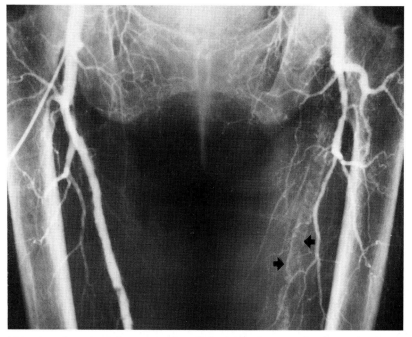

109 Arteriogram: Atheroma and medial calcification. Peripheral vascular disease with atheroma and medial vessel wall calcification can occur as a complication of both long-term dialysis and in patients with renal transplants. On the left there is occlusion of the deep femoral artery with medial wall calcification. On the right there is evidence of diffuse atherosclerosis producing an irregular edge to the contrast in the vessels. Both superficial femoral arteries are also affected by atherosclerosis.

Evaluation of the renal transplant

Renal transplant recipients are prone to many problems, both metabolic and infective. The greatest worry and still the greatest cause of loss of the graft, is the development of irreversible rejection. Obsessional monitoring of graft perfusion, function and drainage, together with repeated cultures from all potential sources and sites of infection, form the basis of care.

Monitoring the graft

Daily plasma creatinine and creatinine clearance are still the best and most reliable arbiters of kidney function. Numerous other tests have been advocated from time to time, but few have stood up to close scrutiny. Perfusion of the graft is usually assessed by renography, and a perfusion index can be calculated from a DTPA renogram (110). Fine needle aspiration biopsy can be carried out, on alternate days if necessary, to monitor the presence or absence of a cellular infiltrate producing rejection (118–121). ^{99m}Tc sulphur colloid can be used to detect rejection in renal transplants. Sulphur colloid is not normally taken up by the kidney, being cleared by the mononuclear phagocytic system of the liver and spleen. During a rejection crisis, the colloid particles become trapped in the rejecting kidney due to the micro-angiopathy associated with rejection. Scanning data and images can be recorded for the first four minutes after injection (vascular phase) and then again at 30 minutes (uptake and trapping). The greater the late uptake the more likely is rejection. Ultrasound can detect rejection but is of particular value in looking for peri-renal collections (blood, urine, lymph or pus). As with the native kidneys, obstruction can be visualised (114). A diagnostic aspiration is readily performed at the time of ultrasound. Table 44 summarises the value of ultrasound.

As the transplant kidney is so accessible, a fine needle can be inserted into the calyces to perform an antegrade pyelogram (111). Although unequivocal evidence of obstruction (e.g. ureteric fibrosis from ischaemia) can be obtained in this way, obstruction may usually be confidently diagnosed by ultrasound, the IVU or ^{99m}Tc DTPA renography.

Arteriography will demonstrate perfusion of the graft, but it is much easier to assess perfusion from a DTPA renogram (110, 115). If there is any doubt, an arteriogram is helpful at showing that the main renal artery and anastomosis are satisfactory (112, 113). Chronic vascular rejection can be revealed by 'pruning' of the smaller vessels within the kidney on arteriography (112). The same information can now be obtained much less invasively using digital subtraction angiography (DSA) (122).

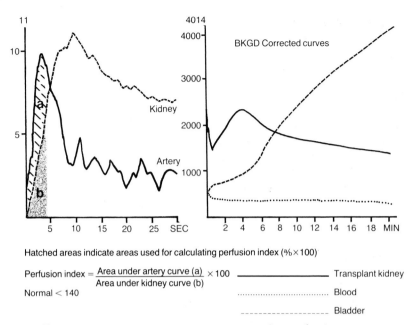

Hatched areas indicate areas used for calculating perfusion index (% × 100)

Perfusion index = $\dfrac{\text{Area under artery curve (a)}}{\text{Area under kidney curve (b)}}$ × 100 —————————— Transplant kidney

Normal < 140 ································· Blood

- - - - - - - - - - - - - - Bladder

110 ^{99m}Tc DTPA Renogram: Perfusion index (renal transplant)

A percutaneous transplant biopsy may be performed readily. As with a biopsy of the native kidney, routine precautions should be taken (see Chapter 6). The transplant biopsy may provide definitive evidence of rejection. It is possible to distinguish three main types of rejection (**123–126**). In addition, a biopsy can provide evidence of recurrence of the original disease or irreversible graft infarction.

Identification of infection
Repeated urine samples, swabs and all drainage fluids, are sent for culture. Pyrexial patients should have blood cultures taken. A weekly chest X-ray is a wise precaution in the first few weeks following transplantation. Viral antibody titres and various rapid culture techniques for the diagnosis of cytomegalo-virus and herpes virus are helpful.

Monitoring the immunosuppressant drugs
If Azathioprine is being used, serial white blood counts and platelet counts are mandatory. A radio-immunoassay for cyclosporin-A is widely available, but blood levels are better monitored using high pressure liquid chromatography. High dose steroids may induce diabetes mellitus, and

regular blood sugar levels and tests of the urine for glucose are obligatory. Liver function tests need to be followed as both Azathioprine and cyclosporin-A, as well as some virus infections, can all disturb the liver.

As yet there is no suitable immunological test that can adequately indicate effective but not excessive immunosuppression. Similarly there is as yet no single reliable test that indicates rejection before tissue damage producing impairment of graft function has occurred.

Table 44: Ultrasound: renal transplant monitoring

Obstruction (dilatation)	Ureteric stenosis:
	Ischaemia
	Rejection
	External compression:
	Haematoma
	Lymphocoele
Collection	Extravasated urine
	Haematoma
	Lymph
	Infection
Rejection criteria:	Increased volume
	Increased cortical thickness
	Increased cortical echoes
	Loss of cortico-medullary differentiation
	Enlargement and squaring off of the pyramids
	Peri-renal halo (extravasated fluid)
	Thinning and reduced echogenecity of the renal sinus

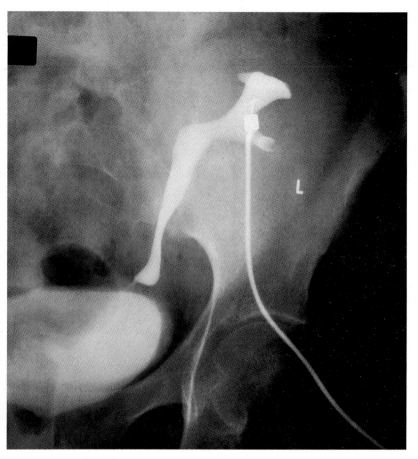

111 Antegrade pyelogram: Renal transplant. This study excludes lower ureteric obstruction which may develop late on post transplant, when an ischaemic stricture can develop. This study was normal.

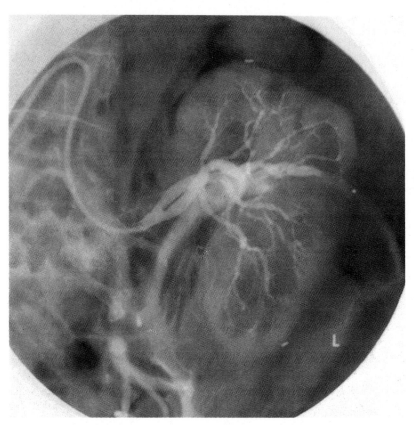

112 Renal arteriogram: Renal transplant. This is a selective transplant arteriogram showing diffuse irregular narrowing of the major intrarenal arteries that can occur with chronic vascular rejection. The catheter has been introduced via the contra-lateral femoral artery to reduce the risk of trauma to the area of the vascular anastomosis.

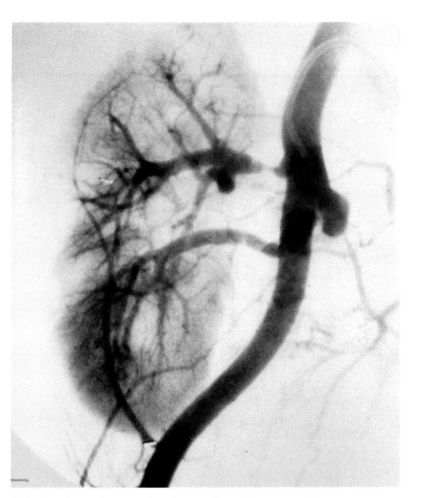

113 Renal arteriogram: Renal transplant. This is a selective arteriogram (subtraction films) showing a tight stenosis of the upper pole artery ın a renal transplant recipient with severe hypertension.

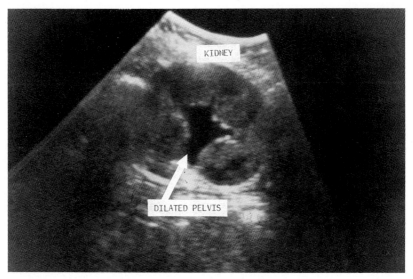

114 Ultrasound: Renal transplant. Obstruction can be diagnosed readily by ultrasound of the transplanted kidney by demonstrating dilatation of the renal pelvis.

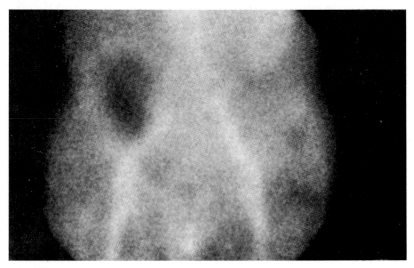

115 ^{99m}Tc DTPA renogram: Graft infarction. Infarction of the renal transplant leaves a 'black hole' of photon deficiency which may be detected on a renogram.

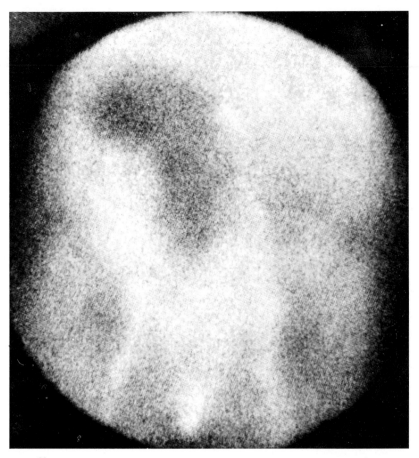

116 ^{99m}Tc DTPA renogram: Peri-renal collection. Reduced background activity around a transplanted kidney ('halo') is produced by a peri-renal collection (e.g. old blood, lymph, pus, etc.) not in direct communication with the circulation.

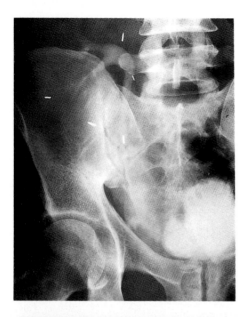

117 IVU: Renal transplant – bladder leak. The edge of the transplanted kidney has been marked by clips at the time of operation. The renal pelvis and ureter are demonstrated, but the striking abnormality is a large leak of contrast from the bladder or vesico-ureteric junction. Surgical repair is often needed in this situation.

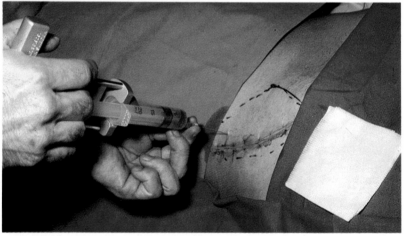

118 Fine needle aspiration biopsy: Method. A 20ml syringe containing about 5ml of tissue culture medium is held in a special syringe holder. After the fine spinal needle (gauge 22) has been inserted in the kidney the syringe holder is squeezed to aspirate a small volume of cells from the graft.

198

119 Fine needle aspiration biopsy: Normal tubular cells have a dark blue cytoplasm. Numerous endothelial cells (eosinophilic) are seen against the background blood (erythrocytes and polymorphs).

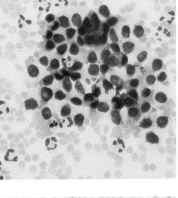

120 Fine needle aspiration biopsy: Acute tubular necrosis is suggested by the vacuolated appearance of the tubular cells' cytoplasm.

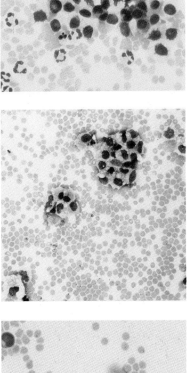

121 Fine needle aspiration biopsy: Acute cellular rejection is indicated by the appearance of lymphocytes, lymphoblasts and in later, more severe rejection episodes, by macrophages.

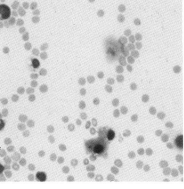

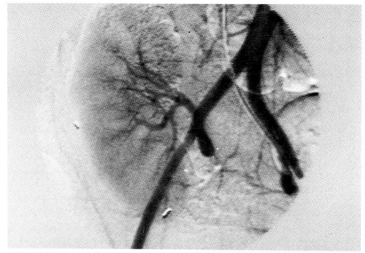

122 DSA in renal transplants:
A: Normal.

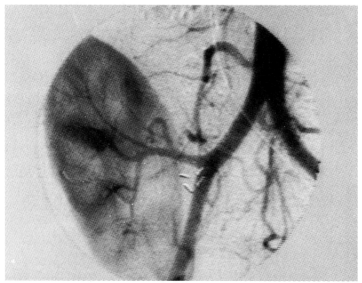

B: Poor graft perfusion due to chronic vascular rejection. Note the peripheral pruning of vessels which do not reach to the edge of the kidney outline.

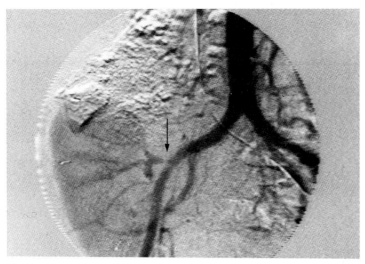

C: Renal artery stenosis (arrow).

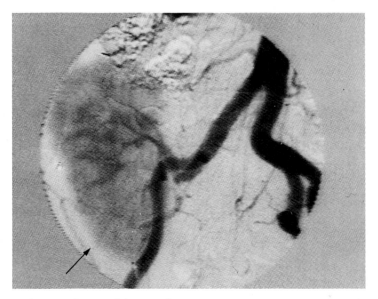

D: Segmental (ventral) hypoperfusion (arrow).

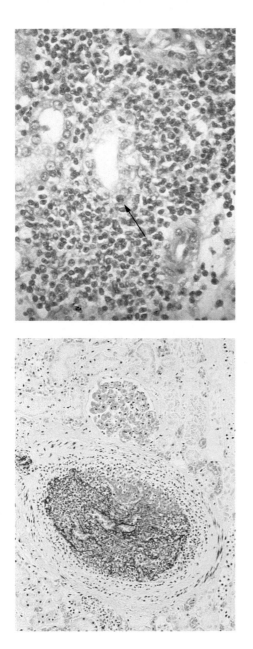

123 Renal transplant biopsy: acute cellular rejection (H&E × 600). This biopsy was taken from a renal transplant during an episode of acute cellular rejection, and stained with haematoxylin and eosin. A dense peritubular inflammatory cell infiltrate of mononuclear cells (lymphocytes, plasma cells and macrophages) separates the remaining tubules. Lymphocytes may be seen between the tubular basement membranes and tubular epithelial cells (tubulitis), as indicated by the arrow.

124 Renal transplant biopsy: Hyperacute rejection (Picro-Mallory × 500). The artery is occluded by thrombus consisting of fibrin, platelets and polymorphs. The tubules appear ghost-like as the result of acute ischaemic necrosis. The glomerulus contains numerous polymorphs and there is stasis in the capillary loops. This type of rejection is seldom seen as it occurs in the presence of pre-formed cytotoxic antibodies. These antibodies should be detected pre-transplant by the leucocyte cross match. Graft nephrectomy is obligatory.

125 Renal transplant biopsy: Vascular rejection (H & E × 500). In addition to an intense mononuclear cell infiltrate around the tubules, this biopsy also shows an oedematous small artery with marked subintimal proliferation, reduplication of the internal elastic lamina and narrowing of the lumen. Treatment is largely ineffective. More chronic changes with subintimal fibrosis may develop months or years after transplantation (see **126**). The lesion is thought to be caused by acquired antibodies to the endothelial cells of vessels.

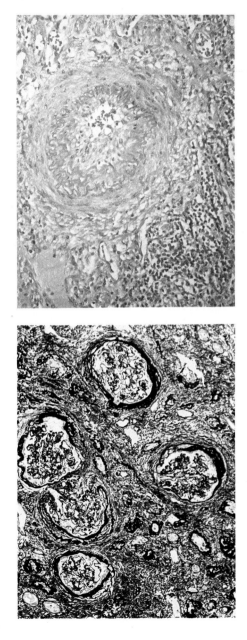

126 Renal transplant biopsy: Chronic vascular rejection (PAMS × 200). There is marked periglomerular fibrosis. The tubular and glomerular basement membranes are collapsed and wrinkled. Tubular atrophy is marked. These appearances are due to ischaemia as a consequence of chronic arterial narrowing developing in lesions like that in **112**.

APPENDIX
I. NORMAL VALUES

Plasma

Osmolality	275 – 295 mOsm/kg	
Sodium	135 – 145 mmol/l	(mEq/l)
Potassium	3.5 – 5 mmol/l	(mEq/l)
Chloride	95 – 105 mmol/l	(mEq/l)
Bicarbonate	24 – 32 mmol/l	(mEq/l)
Anion Gap	6 – 16 mmol/l	(mEq/l)
Magnesium	0.7 – 1 mmol/l	(1.8 – 2.4 mg/dl)
Calcium (total)	2.1 – 2.6 mmol/l	(8.5 – 10.5 mg/dl)
(ionized)	1.135 – 1.32 mmol/l	(4.54 – 5.28 mg/dl)
Phosphate	0.7 – 1.25 mmol/l	(2.1 – 3.9 mg/dl)
B_2 Microglobulin	0.8 – 2.4 mg/l	
Total Protein	60 – 80 g/l	(6 – 8 g/dl)
Albumin	30 – 50 g/l	(3 – 5 g/dl)
Urea	3 – 6.5 mmol/l	(10 – 40 mg/dl)
Creatinine	60 – 120 µmol/l	(0.7 – 1.4 mg/dl)
Uric Acid	0.1 – 0.4 mmol/l	(2 – 7 mg/dl)
Alkaline Phosphatase	3 – 13 KAU	
Hydroxyproline	3 – 21.0 µmol/l	(0.4 – 2.8 mg/l)

Hormones

Plasma Renin Activity = $\begin{cases} \text{Erect: } 1.8 – 6.72 \text{ ng/ml/hr} \\ \text{Supine: } 0.24 – 3.24 \text{ ng/ml/hr} \end{cases}$

Parathyroid Hormone (N terminal) = < 120 pg/ml

(C terminal) = 260 – 1100 pg/ml

$1,25–(OH)_2 D_3$ = 24 – 65 pg/ml

$25 (OH) D_3$ = 5 – 40 ng/ml

$24,25–(OH)_2 D_3$ = 0.5 – 2.5 ng/ml

Anatomical

Measured Kidney Size (bipolar) KUB (IVU) = 12 – 13.5 cm (adults)

$\simeq$ 3 vertebral bodies

Ultrasound = 10 – 12 cm (adults)

Urine

Sodium	100 – 250	mmol/24 hrs.(mEq/24 hrs.)
(depends on diet)		
Potassium	40 – 120	mmol/24 hrs.(mEq/24 hrs.)
(depends on diet)		
Urea	170 – 600	mmol/24 hrs.(10 – 36 g/24 hrs.)
(depends on protein intake)		
Creatinine	9 – 17	mmol/24 hrs.(1 – 2 g/24 hrs.)
Protein	< 250	mg/24 hrs.
Chloride	170 – 250	mmol/24 hrs.(mEq/24 hrs.)
Glucose	< 6	mmol/24 hrs. (< 100 mg/24 hrs.)
Uric Acid	3 – 12	mmol/24 hrs.(0.5 – 2 g/24 hrs.)
Oxalate	30 – 240	μmol/24 hrs. (4 – 30 mg/24 hrs.)
Calcium	2.5 – 7.5	mmol/24 hrs.(100 – 300 mg/24 hrs.)
Phosphate	15 – 50	mmol/24 hrs.(0.5 – 1.5 g/24 hrs.)
Magnesium	2 – 4	mmol/24 hrs.(50 – 100 mg/24 hrs.)

N-Acetyl–β –D– glucosaminidase = 53 – 884 μIU/l/mg creatinine
6 – 134 μIU/l/μmol creatinine
B_2 Microglobulin 30 – 370 μg/24 hrs. (< 25μg/mmol urine creatinine)

Renal Function

GFR (^{51}Cr EDTA)	Males 100 – 150 Females 95 – 125	ml/min/1.73m^2 b.s.a.
ERPF (^{125}I Hippuran)	Males 500 – 600 Females 450 – 650	ml/min/1.73m^2 b.s.a.
Creatinine Clearance	Males 110 – 160 Females 100 – 130	ml/min/1.73m^2 b.s.a.
Urea Clearance	55 – 75	ml/min
Urine Osmolality: range	40 – 1400	mOsm/kg

TUBULAR MAXIMAL REABSORPTION:
Phosphate (TmP) = 3.84 $\pm$ 0.84 mg/min/m^2
Tubular reabsorption of phosphate (TRP) = 85%
Glucose (TmG) = Males 375 $\pm$ 80 mg/min
              Females 303 $\pm$ 55 mg/min
Bicarbonate (Tm HCO$_3$) = 26 mmol/l GFR

THRESHOLDS:
Bicarbonate = 26 mmol/l (mEq/l)
Glucose   = 10 mmol/l (180 mg/dl)
Theoretical Renal Phosphorous Threshold (TRPT) = 2.7 – 4.1 mg/dl.

II. NOMOGRAMS

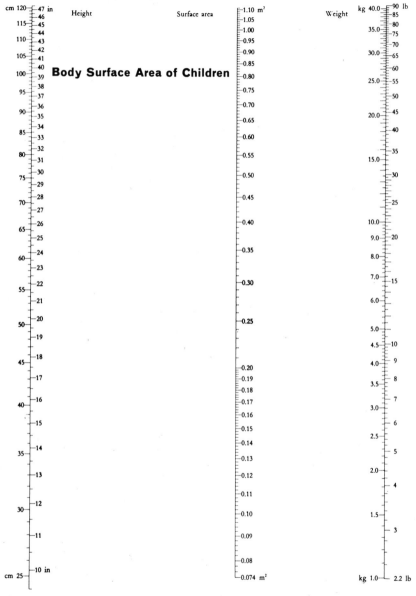

Body Surface Area of Children

cm	Height		Surface area	Weight	kg	lb

Height: cm 120–47 in down to cm 25–10 in

Surface area: 1.10 m² down to 0.074 m²

Weight: kg 40.0–90 lb down to kg 1.0–2.2 lb

206

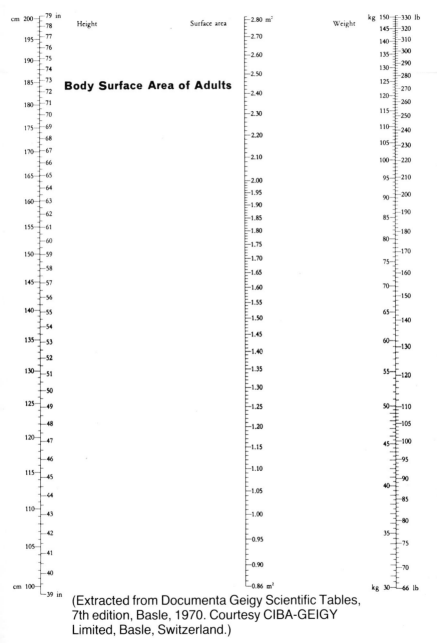

Body Surface Area of Adults

Height	Surface area	Weight

(Extracted from Documenta Geigy Scientific Tables, 7th edition, Basle, 1970. Courtesy CIBA-GEIGY Limited, Basle, Switzerland.)

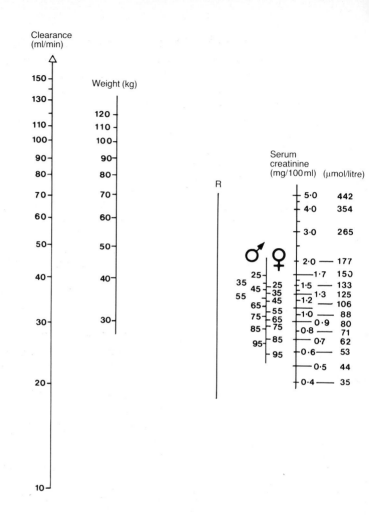

Nomogram for evaluation of the endogenous creatinine clearance.
Use of the nomogram. Connect with a ruler the patient's weight on the second line from the left with the patient's age on the fourth line. Note the point of intersection on *R* and keep the ruler there. Turn the right part of the ruler to the appropriate serum creatinine value and the left side will indicate the clearance in ml/min.

REFERENCES AND FURTHER READING

Barratt, T.M., McLaine, P.N., Soothill, J.F. 1970 *Albumin excretion as a measure of glomerular dysfunction in children.* Arch. Dis. Child. 45 496–501

Bijvoet, O.L.M. and Morgan, B. 1971 *The tubular reabsorption of phosphate in man (TmP/GFR).* In 'Phosphate et métabolisme phosphocalcique'. Ed. D.J. Hioco. 153–180. L'Espansion Scientifique Francaise, Paris.

Birch, D.F., Fairley, K.F., Whitworth, J.A., Forbes, I., Fairley, J.K., Cheshire, G.R., Ryan, G.B. 1983 *Urinary erythrocyte morphology in the diagnosis of glomerular haematuria.* Clin. Nephrol. 20 (2) 78–84.

Boylan, J.W. and Van Liew, J.B. (Eds) 1979 *Symposium on proteinuria and renal protein catabolism.* Kid. Int. 16 (3).

Brody, L.H., Salladay, J.R., Armbruster, K. 1971 *Urinalysis and the urinary sediment.* Med. Clin. North Am. 55 243–266.

Brauman, H. (Ed) 1976 *Fundamentals and clinical aspects of B_2 microglobulin.* Acta Clin. Belg. 31 Suppl 8.

Britton, K.E., Maisey, M.N., Hilson, A.J.W. 1983 *Renal nucleotide studies.* In 'Clinical Nuclear Medicine'. Ed. M.N. Maisey, K.E. Britton, D.L. Gilday. Chapman & Hall, London.

Buffaloe, G.W., Evans, J.E., McIntosh, R.M., Glossock, R.J., Tavel, T.B., Terman, D.S. 1980 *Antibodies to human glomerular basement membrane: modified methodology for detection in human serum.* Clin. Exp. Immunol. 39 136.

Cameron, J.S. and Blandford, G. 1966 *The simple assessment of selectivity in heavy proteinuria.* Lancet II 242–247.

Chantler, C., Garnett, E.S., Parsons, V., Veall, N. 1969 *Glomerular filtration rate measurement in man by the single injection methods using ^{51}Cr EDTA.* Clinical Science 37 169–180.

Dawborn, J.K. 1965 *Application of Heyrovsky's inulin method to automatic analysis.* Clin. Chim. Acta 12 63–66.

Delin, K., Aurell, M., Ewald, J. 1978 *Urinary concentration test with Desmopressin.* Br. Med. J. I (6115) 757–758.

Donckerwolcke, R.A. 1982 *Diagnosis and treatment of renal tubule disorders.* Paed. Clinics N. America 29(4) 895–906.

Duarte C.G. (Editor) 1980 *Renal Function Tests.* Boston, Little, Brown.

Edelmann, C.M., Soriano, J.R., Boichis, H., Gruskin, A.B., Acosta, M. 1967 *Renal bicarbonate reabsorption and hydrogen excretion in normal infants.* J. Clin. Invest. 46 (8) 1309–1317.

Espinel, C.H. 1976 *The FE_{Na} test. Use in the differential diagnosis of acute renal failure.* JAMA 236 (6) 579–581.

Fairley, K.F. and Birch, D.F. 1982 *Haematuria: A simple method for identifying glomerular bleeding.* Kid. Int. 21 (1) 105–108.

Farmer, C.D., Tauxe, W.N., Maher, F.T., Hunt, J.C. 1967 *Measurement of renal function with radio-iodinated diatrizoate and O-iodohippurate.* Am. J. Clin. Path. 47 (1) 9–16.

Focus on Urine Analysis: Oxford. The Medicine Publishing Foundation, 1983.

Foster, P.W., Rick, J.J., Wolfson, W.Q. 1952 *Studies in serum proteins. VI. The extension of the standard Biuret method to the estimation of total protein in urine.* J. Lab. Clin. Med. 39 618–623.

Gadeholt, H. 1964 *Quantitative estimation of urinary sediment with special regard to sources of error.* Brit. Med. J. 1 1547 (o).

Györy, A.Z., Edwards, K.D., Stewart, J.H., Whyte, H.M. 1974 *Comprehensive one-day renal function testing in man.* J. Clin. Path 27 382–391.

Halperin, M.L., Goldstein, M.B., Haig, A. 1974 *Studies on the pathogenesis of type I (distal) renal tubular acidosis as revealed by the urinary PCO_2 tensions.* J. Clin. Invest. 53 669–77.

Häyry, P. and von Willebrand, E. 1981 *Practical guidelines for fine needle aspiration biopsy of human renal allografts.* Ann. Clin. Res. 13 (4–5) 288–3086.

Hendricks, S.N., Lippe, B., Kaplan, S.A., Lee, W.N. 1981 *Differential diagnosis of diabetes insipidus: Use of DDAVP to terminate the seven-hour water deprivation test.* J. Paediatr. 98 (2) 244–6.

Jelliffe, R.W. 1971 *Estimation of creatinine clearance when urine cannot be collected.* Lancet I 975–976.

Kampmann, J., Siersbaek-Nielsen, K., Kristensen, M., Mølholm-Hansen, J. 1974 *Rapid evaluation of creatinine clearance.* Acta Med. Scand. 196 (6) 517–520.

Kunin, C.M., Chesney, R.W., Craig, W.A., England, A.C., De Angelis, C. 1978 *Enzymuria as a marker of renal injury and disease.* Paediatrics 62 751–760.

Kusumi, R.K., Grover, P.J., Kunin, C.M. 1981 *Rapid detection of pyuria by leucocyte esterase activity* JAMA 245 (16) 1653–5.

Lavender, S., Hilton, P.J., Jones, N.F. 1969 *The measurement of glomerular filtration rate in renal disease.* Lancet 2: 1216–1218.

Leaback, D.H. and Walker, P.G. 1961 *Studies on glucosaminidase: 4. The fluorimetric assay of N-acetyl-B-glucosaminidase.* Biochemical Journal 78 151–156.

Lubec, G. (Ed) 1983 *Non-invasive diagnosis of kidney disease.* Basel, New York: Karger.

Monson, J.P. and Richards, P. 1978 *Desmopressin urine concentration test.* Br. Med. J. I (6104) 24.

Pak, C.Y., Kaplan, R., Bone, H., Townsend, J., Waters, O. 1975 *A simple test for the diagnosis of absorptive, resorptive and renal hypercalcuria.* N. Eng. J. Med. 292. 497–500.

Pitts, R.F., 1963 *Physiology of the kidney and body fluids.* Year Book Medical Publishers Incorporated, Chicago.

Rosenthal, A.F. and Yaseen, A. 1969 *Improved qualitative screening test for cystinuria and homocystinuria.* Clin. Chim. Acta 26 363–364.

Schrier, R.W. (Ed) *Renal and electrolyte disorders.* 2nd Edition 1980, Little, Brown.

Schnurr, E. 1983 *Inulin and PAH clearance in the steady state without urine collection.* Chapter 5 75–84. In 'Non-Invasive Diagnosis of Kidney Disease'. Ed. G. Lubec. Basel, New York: Karger.

Sherwood, T., Davidson, A.J., Talner, L.B. 1980 *Uroradiology.* Blackwell Scientific Publications.

Smith, H.W. 1956 *Principles of Renal Physiology.* Oxford University Press, New York.

Stamp, T.C. and Stacey, T.E. 1970 *Evaluation of theoretical renal phosphorus threshold as an index of renal phosphorus handling.* Clin. Science 39 505–516.

Thomsen, K., and Schon, M. 1968 *Renal lithium excretion in man.* AM. J. Physiol. 215 (4) 823–827.

Tucker, S.M., Boyd, P.J., Thompson, A.E., Price, R.G. 1975 *Automated assay of N-acetyl-β-glucosaminidase in normal and pathological human urine.* Clin. Chim. Acta 62 (2) 333–339.

Wagoner, R.D., Tauxe, W.N., Maher, F.T., Hunt, J.C. 1964 *Measurement of effective renal plasma flow with sodium iodohippurate [131]I.* JAMA 187 (11) 811–813.

de Wardener, H.E. 1973 *The kidney: an outline of normal and abnormal structure and function.* 4th Edition. Churchill Livingstone, Edinburgh and London.

Watts, R.W.E., Mitchell, F.L., Veall, N. 1972 *Renal function tests suitable for clinical practice.* Clinical Review No. 2 9 (1) 3–18.

Wrong, O. and Davis, H.E.F. 1959 *The excretion of acid in renal disease.* Quart. J. Med. 28 259–313.

Index